EBOLA'S
EVOLUTION

EBOLA'S EVOLUTION

TURNING DESPAIR TO DELIVERANCE: A ROAD MAP FOR COVID-19

MICHAEL B.A. OLDSTONE *and*
MADELEINE ROSE OLDSTONE

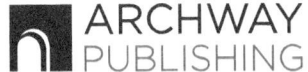

Archway Publishing books may be ordered through booksellers or by contacting:

Archway Publishing
1663 Liberty Drive
Bloomington, IN 47403
www.archwaypublishing.com
844-669-3957

ISBN: 978-1-6657-0248-5 (sc)
ISBN: 978-1-6657-0247-8 (hc)
ISBN: 978-1-6657-0249-2 (e)

Library of Congress Control Number: 2021902089

Print information available on the last page.

Archway Publishing rev. date: 05/25/2021

"Emerging infectious diseases…remain the major cause of death worldwide and will not be conquered during our lifetimes…despite many potential defenses -- vaccines, antibiotics, diagnostic tools -- we are intrinsically more vulnerable than before, at least in terms of pandemics and communicable diseases."

Joshua Lederberg
1958 Nobel Laureate in Medicine

"We exist in a Darwin-like survival battle against the advancement, mutation and selection of previous, new and evolving viruses (think Ebola, Influenza, HIV, COVID-19) opposed and countered only by our fortitude, intelligence and technical advances."

Michael B. A. Oldstone

DEDICATION

This book is dedicated to those physicians, nurses, and health care workers, native and foreign who combatted Ebola virus outbreaks in West Africa (2013-2016) and Central Africa (2018-2020) . Especially to the staff and workers at the Kenema Government Hospital in West Africa, Sheik Humar Khan, Pardis Sabeti, Robert Garry, and many of whom lost their lives in the battle to engage and control Ebola, to Doctors Without Borders, and all those who personally confronted Ebola since its initial onset in Central Africa and continue to do so, well represent the following words:

No man is an island,
Entire of itself.
Each is a piece of the continent,
A part of the main.
If a clod be washed away by the sea,
Europe is the less.
As well as if a promontory were.
As well as if a manor of thine own
Or of thine friend's were.
Each man's death diminishes me,
For I am involved in mankind.
Therefore, send not to know
For whom the bell tolls,
It tolls for thee.

John Donne
1624

Michael B.A. Oldstone is professor emeritus at The Scripps Research Institute where he developed and directed the laboratory of viral immunobiology for four decades. He is an elected member of the National Academy of Sciences and the National Academy of Medicine, the recipient of numerous scientific honors and elections to scientific societies nationally and internationally. He was a member of the SAGE executive board of the World Health Organization (WHO), a consultant to the WHO for the eradication of poliomyelitis and measles and scientific reviewer for the National Institutes of Health (NIH).

Madeleine Rose Oldstone graduated from the College of Diplomacy at Seton Hall University and received a master's degree from American University's School of Public Affairs in Public Policy. Her interest and commitment are to world health problems, policy, and diplomacy.

ACKNOWLEDGMENTS

The authors thank Drs. Robert Garry, Pardis Sabeti, and Kristian Andersen for their input regarding the Ebola 2013-2016 outbreak in Sierra Leone and in Kenema Government Hospital. We are also grateful to the staff of Kenema Government Hospital and Dr. Brian Sullivan for providing insights. We received input and unpublished data on use and results for the Ebola vaccine in 2018-2020 outbreak at Democratic Republic of the Congo courtesy of Drs. Beth Ann Griswold-Collier Executive Director of Vaccines Clinical Research and Roger Perlmutter President of Merck Research Laboratories. Robert Garry for insights and discussion of the 2018-2020 Ebola outbreak in the Congo. We thank Pardis Sabeti, Brian Sullivan, and Kristian Andersen for providing photographs used in this book, and Janet Hightower for coupling the photographs into figures and for design of the book's cover. We also acknowledge Gay Wilkins-Blade (TSRI), my faithful assistant of over three decades who typed and retyped our manuscript. We thank Phyllis Minick, our editor in La Jolla, for insights and suggestions.

AUTHOR'S NOTE
EBOLA as a road map for COVID-19

Ebola, first detected in 1976 in the Democratic Republic of the Congo (formerly named Zaire), and Covid-19, first identified in China in late 2019 share several traits. Both Ebola and Covid-19 infections elicit fear, show no remorse or distinction to the various social classes they infect, and kill. Both are equal opportunity killers. They destroy the social fabric of society, cause severe economic hardship, and with ease cross local, national, and international borders. These two pathogens that cause Ebola and Covid-19 are RNA viruses. RNA viruses frequently mutate as they lack or have a poor machinery in place to filter out the many mutants they generate. Mutant viruses then survive (or not) according to their fitness and selection to emerge as new swarms of virus particles (quasi-species). Some of these newly produced viruses may then gain an enhanced ability to spread, become more harmful, or better able to escape immune surveillance. Ebola and Covid-19 viruses cause enough infections to overwhelm populations and compromise health care systems.

These two viruses also differ distinctly. Ebola virus primarily occupies rural areas in Africa but has reached cities, other continents and countries. Covid-19 virus also leaves its mark in rural and urban Africa but is heavily present in rural and metropolitan areas throughout the world in major cities like New York, Paris, Berlin, Tokyo, and a long list of others. The mortality rates also differ greatly by geography and timing. Infection with Ebola virus, in the 18 outbreaks since 1976, lead to a mortality rate of 30%-89% with an average of 63%. Usually 200 to 400 individuals in rural settings are infected. However, during two recent outbreaks over 28,000 persons in the West African scourge of 2013-2016 and over 2,500 in the Democratic

Republic of the Congo during 2018-2020 were infected. By contrast, Covid-19 has infected millions since its initial 10 months of discovery. Covid-19 is spread by the respiratory route, the most favorable way to transmit a virus to the largest available population segment, whereas Ebola spreads by contact via touching infected persons or handling their utensils, linen or fluids (sweat, tears, blood, etc.) and is less aggressively passed. However, one strain of Ebola, Ebola Reston, a less virulent strain, can be transmitted by the aerosol route from one non-human primate to others. According to serologic evidence Ebola Reston has been transmitted from non-human primates to humans in monkey holding facilities. The handlers were asymptomatic or had mild symptoms. Yet, the Reston Ebola virus theoretically could mutate to a more virulent form and possess the ability for better spread to the human population; if so, watch out for a nightmare scenario.

In fact, universal despair was been the common response to both Ebola and Covid-19 infections. Despair marked experiences with Ebola and Covid-19 viruses because there were no effective anti-viral therapies to control the acute infection or a vaccine to inhibit the spread of either virus. Only recently, in 2019, did a measure of deliverance come to those acutely infected with Ebola virus. Deliverance arrived in the form of several candidate anti-Ebola viral drugs manufactured in sufficient amounts to have undergone clinical safety trials. Under extraordinarily difficult conditions, four candidate drugs were administrated for effectiveness in Africa during an Ebola outbreak. Impressively, two of the four drugs displayed a significant ability to treat the acute infection and successfully reduce morbidity and mortality. As for Covid-19 infection, no such therapy for the acute early phase of infection is yet on hand. However, the same advanced technologies that successfully generated anti-Ebola virus drugs are being followed to create anti-Covid-19 therapeutics. Importantly of the four anti-Ebola drugs evaluated, all had showed significant protective value in non-human primates infected with Ebola virus. Only two of the four were effective in humans. Clearly, time is required to screen drugs for effectiveness because those that work in non-human primates may not do so in humans. Therein lies a lesson for Covid-19.

Deliverance for helplessness with Ebola virus infection also came from the development of a vaccine that significantly arrested the spread of Ebola virus to uninfected individuals. This vaccine was first tested in 2014 during the Ebola virus outbreak to prevent its spread to individuals in Liberia in West Africa. However, the vaccine's effectiveness remained controversial until the outbreak in 2018-2020 in the Democratic Republic of the Congo settled the issue. A clinical trial confirmed that the vaccine significantly interrupted the spread of Ebola infection. The bottom-line outcome was that effective anti-Ebola virus drugs became available to treat infected patients in the acute stage of disease and an effective vaccine successfully inhibited the viral spread. Therapeutic breakthroughs that were not possible just a few years ago are now available. It is likely that a similar scenario will manage Covid-19 infection.

This book characterizes the Ebola virus and the infection it causes. The despair accompanying this infection arose from repeated outbreaks over forty years with one of the most lethal viruses known to humans. The focus is on the 2013-2016 outbreak in Sierra Leone, primarily at the Kenema Government Hospital (KGH), where one of the author's (Michael Oldstone) laboratory staff was present. Here we unlock the mysteries of the largest outbreaks of one of the world's most fearsome viruses.

What is Ebola? Why did this plague emerge? How did anti-viral therapies and a vaccine arise? Does this experience with Ebola provide a road map for navigating Covid-19? This book answers those questions, while introducing fascinating people thrust into a situation as dramatic as that could be imagined in a blockbuster novel or movie. We record in sequence and detective-story style how the initial outbreak of Ebola in West Africa traveled from the index case in rural Guinea to

Sierra Leone and recount the work and fate of those working at the KGH isolation ward in Sierra Leone. The book provides vignettes of the three major players involved with Ebola at KGH: Sheik Humar Khan, Pardis Sabeti, and Robert Garry, and emphasizes the poor preparation and negligible understanding of Ebola virus, its spread and the infected host's immune response. The inadequate response of governments whose citizens were infected, from the WHO and others as well as poor financial assistance by non-government organizations (NGO) and other countries allowed the enhanced spread, killing, and devastation in countries where Ebola flourished. Solutions to correct these deficiencies for future epidemics/pandemics are presented. How such deficiencies were or were not corrected are compared when two years after the first major onset the second largest Ebola outbreak occurred. The rapid search, field testing, availability and use of the first successful anti-Ebola drugs and a vaccine are presented. The problems of incompetence, politics trumping science, citizen unrest, failure to accept public health measures, and unpreparedness for these Ebola outbreaks share much in common with the current Covid-19 pandemic.

By reading this book you will come to understand why the world was unprepared for the outbreak of such a deadly pathogen as Ebola virus and why, as is obvious, it still lacks solutions for other pandemics like Covid-19. You will gain intimate knowledge of a pathogen that spread like a hurricane over a region of the world that lacked the resources and knowledge to fight it. After meeting people here who fought with the limited resources on hand and became heroes by putting the possibility of saving their patients ahead of protecting their own lives, in the end, you will gain insights into steps that must be taken to ensure that the present horrific virus outbreaks like Ebola and Covid-19 are controlled and never arise again anywhere in the world.

FOREWORD

Robert Garry

Ebola's Evolution, a timely, needed and well-presented book by Michael Oldstone and Madeleine Rose Oldstone, unlocks the mysteries of the largest two outbreaks of one of the world's most fearsome viruses. What is Ebola? Why did this happen? Here you will find the answers to these questions, while meeting fascinating people thrust into a situation as dramatic as any that could be imagined in a blockbuster novel or movie.

By reading this book you will come to understand why the world was unprepared for the outbreak of such a deadly pathogen as Ebola virus, it still is and recent attempts to tame Ebola. You will gain intimate knowledge of a pathogen that spread like a tsunami over a region of the world that lacked the resources to fight it and beyond. You will meet a group of people (me among them) that by chance were already there to fight another deadly virus. You will find out how in a matter of weeks this small group of doctors, nurses and scientists were overwhelmed and why these matters. You will meet people that fought with limited resources at hand and became heroes that put the possibility of saving their patients ahead of their own lives. In the end you will gain insights into steps that must be taken to ensure that such a horrific virus outbreak never happens again anywhere in the world.

This book exists because Michael Oldstone is passionate about viruses. Michael has devoted his career to understanding how viruses undermine and manipulate the immune system thereby causing disease. His investigations of lymphocytic choriomeningitis virus, easier known as LCMV, have been beacons shining the light of understanding about fundamental concepts of infectious diseases. LCMV infects the common house mouse around the world; its cousin Lassa virus causes a severe disease known as Lassa fever in humans living in Sierra Leone, Nigeria and other parts of West Africa. Ebola and Lassa fever are so similar that even an experienced doctor cannot tell if a patient has one disease or the other. Unlike Ebola, however, Lassa fever does not cause outbreaks, but is continuously erupting usually in small disease clusters. There is another difference. Lassa fever is somewhat less contagious than Ebola. It does not spread as easily from person to person. Until the outbreak in West Africa the full explosive potential of Ebola had not yet been felt.

In late 2013 I had the privilege of working with Michael to develop a proposal to the National Institutes of Health to apply lessons learned about LCMV infection in mice to Lassa fever in humans. Little was known about how Lassa virus undercuts human immunity. Particularly sparse was knowledge in Michael's specialty known as T cell immunity. Patients from across Sierra Leone come all year round to the Lassa fever ward in Kenema, which is located near the borders of Guinea and Liberia. Our team had been working on Lassa fever in Kenema for over a decade. Our new plan was to use the tools Michael had developed over decades of study of LCMV to probe T cell immunity to Lassa virus in humans. As 2013 ended, we did not know that only a few hours drive away Ebola had just begun to spread to people, and that everything would change.

I will close this brief Introduction by noting a fortuitous circumstance that has produced a boon for readers of this book. As it turns out, the only aspect of his life more precious than science to Michael Oldstone is his family. Teaming this eminent scientist (if there were to be a Wikipedia entry for "eminent scientist" Michael Oldstone's picture could surely appear beside it as one of the best examples) with his nonscientist granddaughter ensured that **Ebola's Evolution** is devoid of unexplained jargon and inaccessible technical language. Rather, you have before you a real-life drama about a virus that both terrorized and fascinated the world told in a style that flows seamlessly, teaches without being pedantic, and entertains immensely. What follows is the definitive account of the deadliest outbreak of Ebola.

Robert Garry
Tulane University
Program Manager, Viral Hemorrhagic Fever Consortium
New Orleans

INTRODUCTION

West Africa - July 2014

The light in Sierra Leone's midafternoon heat, then progressive, intermittent darkness encompassed Sheik Humar Khan. Khan was wracked with fever, pain, sweating, continued diarrhea, and increasing difficulty in keeping his eyes open. Sheik Khan, the best known physician studying and treating viral hemorrhagic diseases in Sierra Leone and well recognized internationally, headed the Kenema Government Hospital (KGH).[1] This small hospital was over-flooded with Ebola-infected patients. All beds and even open spaces, including floors, contained sick individuals, many vomiting and oozing blood potentially spreading virus until they died. Fewer than half of the hospitalized patients recovered. The hospital staff was overwhelmed and exhausted, caring for more than 80 patients in a 14-bed facility dedicated to viral hemorrhagic fevers. Other sick patients were lying outside on the hospital grounds. Khan worked 16 to 18 hours a day. His family warned him to leave this center of Ebola misery. But he told his sister, "If I leave, then who will come and fill my shoes."[2] Already the hospital's head nurse, Mballu Fonnie, and multiple members of the hospital health staff had died. In areas surrounding the hospital, whispers spread that people go in but don't come out alive. Now, after the testing of Sheik Khan's blood confirmed a diagnosis of Ebola virus infection, he was concerned that his illness would further demoralize KGH's staff and frighten their patients. Khan worried for his life, "I'm afraid for my life, because I cherish my life. And if you are afraid then you must take the maximum precautions, stay vigilant and stay on your guard."[1] As evening darkened, Khan was taken from his bed, moved into a vehicle, and driven along dirt roads to Kailahun district in eastern Sierra Leone, 75 miles away, where Doctors Without Borders had set up an Ebola care center. There, after initial stabilization, Khan's medical condition began a rapid decline. The therapy available was fluids to replace the 6-10 liters he had already lost by diarrhea, vomiting, and sweating. A potential alternative, an anti-Ebola antibody (protein made against the Ebola virus) called ZMapp, stored at this Doctors Without Borders center, but never used for treating humans. In a previous experimental study, ZMapp had been effective in treating Ebola in monkeys, even when provided five days into their illness, but its effect on humans was completely unchartered.[3] Nevertheless, Khan was dying as were many natives, local health care workers as well as health care professionals and others from Western countries.

At the Doctors Without Borders center where Khan now awaited help were others infected with Ebola and also gravely sick. The center had barely enough ZMapp for three or four persons. The choice of which patients received ZMapp lay primarily in the hands of a team at the Canadian company that made ZMapp and members of Doctors Without Borders at the Kailahun treatment center. Also involved were representatives from the World Health Organization, United States Communicable Disease Center, and National Institutes of Health. Sheik Khan was not told that ZMapp was available. The health officials deliberated while considering that neither the antibody's therapeutic effectiveness nor its side effects were known. In the end, they decided not to tell Khan about ZMapp or if it could be used on him. Instead, the ZMapp was transported to Guinea where two Ebola-infected victims were treated: a volunteer American physician, Kent Brantly, and a volunteer American health worker, Nancy Writebol, both from Samaritan's Purse charity. Later a priest, Miguel Pajares, from Spain was also given ZMapp. The first two survived but the priest died.[4]

Khan's condition worsened. He reflected on his life of

wanting to be a physician and contribute to his country's health, his training in Sierra Leone Medical School, medical residency, a rapid ascent as a physician and expert in therapeutics, his many collaborators from the West, especially Pardis Sabeti from The Broad Institute at MIT and Harvard, and Robert Garry and colleagues from the Tulane Medical School.[5] He thought of his work in treating those in need, the good life he had, and whether there was a good death. Then Khan's eyes got heavier; no longer could he open them, and he died. Sheik Khan, who treated over 100 Ebola patients at KGH since the first one entered in March, fell ill in mid-July and tested positive for Ebola at KGH on 22 July, traveled to Kailahun and died 29 July at the Doctors Without Borders treatment center.[6]

Central Africa: Democratic Republic of the Congo (DRC) - March 2020

In addition to Sheik Humar Khan, by the end of the Ebola outbreak in West Africa, 28,616 individuals had been infected and 11,310 died, representing the largest outbreak of this viral infection. Then in the northeastern part of the DRC the second largest outbreak occurred.[7] This outbreak ended in March 2020 involving 3,463 verified infectious cases and 2,280 deaths. The two year time interval between 2013-2016 and 2018-2020 allowed for assessment of problems and formation of corrections of many deficiencies noted in patient care, protection of health care workers, establishing and having protocols in place to test the effectiveness of ZMapp and three other anti-viral therapeutic drugs during the Ebola virus infection. In addition, an anti-Ebola vaccine was sufficiently field tested to determine its effectiveness to prevent or minimize Ebola virus infection. Thus, the two years between 2016 and 2018 were not wasted in terms of preparation of potential anti-Ebola virus therapies, enhanced patient care and insights to better protect health care workers.

This book recalls the origin of Ebola, a relatively new infectious disease, first demonstrated in 1976 in Central Africa, and records the focal outbreaks throughout Central Africa from 1976 until 2016. However, the book's emphasis is the 2013-2016 West African outbreak where Ebola first appeared as an unknown "mysterious infectious disease" in the village of Meliandou in Guinea and spread from there to Sierra Leone and Liberia. The infection and death rates of the single 2013-2016 West African outbreak exceeded the accumulated infections and deaths in total of the previous 25 Ebola outbreaks in Central Africa. The outbreak and spread in Sierra Leone consumed the majority of Ebola cases in West Africa. In Sierra Leone teams of health care workers, virologists, immunologists, and geneticists at Kenema and KGH were on the front line and their personal stress and comments form a large part of the body of this book. Sheik Humar Khan, a native of Sierra Leone, was head of the clinical Viral Hemorrhagic Program, Pardis Sabeti of The Broad Institute of MIT and Harvard, and Robert Garry of Tulane Medical School were the other leading participants, and along with their colleagues entered in the fight to diagnose, treat, and understand the Ebola outbreak. Pardis Sabeti, a M.D. and geneticist, and her colleagues analyzed the evolution of the Ebola virus as it spread from patient to patient and within the individual patient. Robert Garry was the program director and organizer for research at KGH, in conjunction with the Sierra Leone Ministry of Health and Sanitation. The personal experiences of these individuals, their highs and lows, run through this book as do the medical catastrophes and economic hardships resulting from Ebola. The story would not be complete without pointing to the heroes and their accomplishments on one side of the coin, and the errors, mismanagement and those responsible for prolonging the terror of Ebola on the other side of the coin. An assessment of errors made locally and internationally was necessary so a similar disaster to that of Ebola 2013-2016 in West Africa would be better controlled. The corrections made and strides in therapeutic intervention during the 2018-2020 outbreak is critiqued and problems still existing is illuminated in this book. Lastly, this book recognizes and grieves for the over 11,000 deaths in West Africa and over 2,200 deaths in Central Africa, as well as the 40% of the 1,000+ health care providers who gave their lives in the fight to contain Ebola including Sheik Humar Khan.

Michael B.A. Oldstone
Madeleine Rose Oldstone
The Scripps Research Institute
Washington, D.C.
La Jolla, California

CONTENTS

Ebola's Origin: A Limited but Devastating Viral Hemorrhagic Disease of Central Africa

The name Ebola comes from a corruption of the French word for the river Legbala (as named in the Ngbandi language). This river is the head stream of the Mongala River, a tributary of the Congo River approximately 166 miles long, in the northern part of the Democratic Republic of the Congo (DRC). This former part of the Belgian Congo was then known as Zaire. In 1976, infection by the so-called Ebola virus was first identified in the town of Yambuku,[1] located 60 miles from the Ebola River. Rather than stigmatize Yambuku by naming the virus after the town, and thus hamper its economy or reputation, Dr. Peter Piot, now Director of the London School of Hygiene and Tropical Medicine, called the virus by the river's name. This politically correct technique had been in use earlier for naming, as shown by the outbreak of Hantavirus infection, occurring in the Four-Corners region of the United States where Colorado borders New Mexico, Utah, and Arizona.[1] Originally named Hanta Four-Corners virus, which depicted the geographic site where the virus was found, after disapproval by merchants and residents in the area, the pathogen underwent a change of name to Sin Nombre virus (Spanish for no-name virus) to avoid political and economic outfall.[2] Thus Ebola virus, like Sin Nombre virus, joins the list of politically correct viruses.

In the first outbreak of Ebola virus infections, 318 victims were identified, of whom 279 died, a mortality of 88%.[1,3] This virus was christened Ebola Zaire, basically the same virus strain that caused the two largest recent outbreaks one in West Africa in 2013-2016[3] and one in Central Africa 2018-2020. Since 1976, all outbreaks of Ebola virus infection have occurred in Central Africa (Zaire, Sudan, Kenya, Gabon, and Uganda) except for the 2013-2016 occurrences in Guinea, Liberia, and Sierra Leone, and that of one person in the Ivory Coast, West Africa in 1994.[3-6] That person was a scientist who became infected after doing an autopsy on a chimpanzee found in the Taï Forest. It is believed that Ebola was derived from the infected chimpanzee's blood.[5,6] The Taï Forest is a national park in Cote d'Ivorie containing one of the last areas of primary rainforest in West Africa.[7] The national park was created in 1926 and promoted as a national park in 1972. In 1982, it was declared a World Heritage Site owing to the breadth of its flora and fauna; five mammalian species in the forest (pygmy hippopotamus, olive colobus monkeys, leopards, chimpanzees, and Jentink's duiker) are on the Red List of threatened species. This forest is approximately 100km from the Ivorian coast on the border of Liberia between the Cavalla and Sassandra Rivers. The size of the park is 4,540 km and altitudes vary from 80m to 396m. As its name implies, the Taï Forest Ebola virus strain is believed to have originated at this site[3,1], presumably a natural reservoir of the Ebola virus. This is the likely area from which the 2013 Ebola outbreak occurred before spreading through Guinea, Sierra Leone, and Liberia in West Africa during 2013-2016. None of the multiple occurrences in Central Africa before the 2018-2020 Kivu outbreak, including the original 1976 outbreak, affected more than 425 individuals or caused more than 280 deaths (Figure 1).[3,6,8] Yet, by contrast, the 25th outbreak of Ebola in 2013-2016 in northwestern Africa infected over 28,000 people and killed over 11,000. How this happened, whether the viruses, people or environments differed, and whether the infection could have been controlled are the subjects of this book along with a description of the epidemic.

The 1976 eruption of Ebola in Zaire, Central Africa, provided lessons for how to control future outbreaks of this disease. Unfortunately, not all those lessons were learned or sufficiently applied to control the 2013-2016 Ebola outbreak that devastated Guinea, Liberia, and Sierra Leone in West Africa and the 2018-2020 outbreak in Central Africa. Yet the Ebola virus that appeared in the first outbreak (called Ebola Zaire) is basically the same virus found in West Africa in 2013-2016[4] and the 2018-2020 outbreak in Central Africa. So what are the lessons and their consequences for those afflicted in the future?[9]

The year 1976 marked the first recorded case of an Ebola virus infection. The index person was treated at Yambuku Mission Hospital for nosebleed and diarrhea, then fever and lethargy, systemic symptoms that resembled common regional diseases such as malaria, yellow fever, and typhoid fever. This index patient came from a rural area and, though not proven, likely became infected initially after hunting and preparing food contaminated by the blood or saliva of an Ebola-infected monkey or fruit bat. Even when fruit bats carry Ebola virus, they can be clinically healthy and show no signs or symptoms of infection. Infected monkeys usually become ill and die; fruit bats do not. The Yambuku Mission Hospital had 120 beds, and the Ebola virus infection spread rapidly from the single index case to other patients in the hospital via use of unsterilized needles, syringes, scissors, and other instruments. At that time and place, hospital instruments were cleaned by simply washing and then rinsing with distilled water before reuse. The virus then spread to not only other patients but also health care workers exposed to blood and body fluids from infected patients. Blood, body fluids, saliva, and tears are now known to contain large amounts of infectious Ebola virus. Of the Yambuku Mission Hospital's 17 staff members, 13 became sick, and 11 died. Health care workers and ill patients infected visitors who then transmitted the infection to family members and others on return to their villages. Thus, from the single index case, 318 people became infected, and 280 died. The hospital closed when the medical director and three Belgian missionaries died. Many infected individuals and their contacts fled to their home villages out of fear of disease and suspicion of the non-functioning Western medical system. Those fleeing often sought traditional therapies from native health healers.[3]

Concurrently, the government of Zaire contacted the United States Centers for Disease Control (CDC) in Atlanta, Georgia, for assistance. Zaire's officials planned to join with and assist a group of international scientists and health care workers to elucidate and control this outbreak of a lethal hemorrhagic fever of unknown origin. The Zaire government of President Mobutu Sese Seko and his Council of Ministers, with the minister of health and the international community, shared information and had daily or frequent meetings. More than 70 health care workers were assigned to the field for surveillance and education. The government attempted to quarantine 275,000 people in the area and prohibited commercial plane and boat traffic. Orders were distributed that no one was to leave the villages, and no strangers were allowed to enter them. Four-person teams for health care surveillance, most often led by a physician or nurse, were trained to recognize Ebola hemorrhagic disease. A diagnostic test for Ebola was developed. These knowledgeable surveillance teams visited over 550 villages at least twice over a two-month period, and a third time for the 55 villages where Ebola had been found.

Of great importance were their meetings with the elders and chiefs who headed these villages to impart knowledge about the disease. Team members spoke about the infection's spread and containment, the need to avoid contact with sick individuals, and what burial procedure was safe to follow. In many villages, sick patients were placed in outlying huts, following a common practice used earlier for isolation of individuals with smallpox. One family member brought food and water to the isolation hut. When the patient died, the traditional rite of washing and touching the body by family and friends was discouraged. Dead bodies were covered with bleach disinfectant, wrapped in shrouds and buried. Isolation huts housing those who died and their garments were burned.

Hence, the lessons learned were: 1) The first signs of disease were diarrhea, fever, and lethargy. However, these signs and symptoms were often confused with those of other febrile illnesses like typhoid fever, yellow fever, malaria. 2) Infected natives frequently emerged from rural areas then came or were brought to care centers. 3) Transmission occurred by direct contact with infected individuals' blood and body fluids, and spread was amplified by poor hospital practices such as reusing needles and inadequately isolating the sick. Hospital care workers were especially vulnerable and needed protective clothing and adequate health care help. 4) Education and compassion were required to overcome the fear of infection and disease. Training emphasized the important of isolation and absolute necessity to disregard the usual cultural traditions of touching and washing the body of a deceased family member or friend. 5) The involvement of both local and central governments along with international cooperation was obligatory. 6) Formation of health care surveillance groups to monitor local and rural populations was required. 7) Since attempts to physically blockade the migration of people were not effective, as fleeing individuals managed to escape through all barriers erected, the need for education was emphasized repeatedly. 8) Further established were the facts that infection from needle sticks required an incubation period of 6 days for symptoms to appear; and person-to-person contact took a mean of 8 days with a range of 1 to 21 days; therefore, a mandatory quarantine period of 42 days (double 21 days) was selected to prevent further contamination.[3,5,9]

Two years later, in 1978, Ebola resurfaced at Tandala Mission Hospital, located about 155 miles from Yambuku. In this instance, the disease did not spread. The physician in charge, who had participated in the Yambuku outbreak, suspected that the agent of infection was Ebola virus and isolated the 9-year-old girl who came from a rural village to enter the hospital. Only one other person became infected with Ebola virus, the girl's younger sister.

However, an extraordinary challenge in the control of Ebola was to occur seven years later in 1995. That year's outbreak provided the stringent test of whether the lessons of containment were not only learned but could also be applied to stop a devastating spread of the infection into the largest population center in the country recently renamed from Zaire to the Democratic Republic of the Congo (DRC). The Kikwit General Hospital in DRC was separated from the capital city by 217 miles and 5 hours driving time along well-traveled roads. In Kinshasa, the capital, lived several million susceptible individuals, many in close quarters and in slums.

After lying quiescent in DRC (Zaire) for 18 years and for 16 years elsewhere in central Africa (Sudan in 1979 infecting 34 individuals with a mortality rate of 65%), Ebola reappeared in DRC in May 1995. Increasing numbers of patients sick with hemorrhagic fever entered the Kikwit General Hospital.[3] In short order, many of the patients hospitalized for treatment, their families who accompanied them, and many nurses and doctors who treated those sick individuals died. Ebola had been suspected by local physicians who observed similar cases 19 years earlier. As recorded …"When a 36-year-old lab technician known as Kinfumu checked into the general hospital in Kikwit, Zaire, last month, complaining of diarrhea and a fever, anyone could have mistaken his illness for the dysentery that was plaguing the city. Nurses, doctors, and nuns did what they could to help the young man. They soon saw that this disease wasn't just dysentery. Blood began oozing from orifices in his body. Within four days he was dead. By then the illness had all but liquefied his internal organs.[10]

That was just the beginning. The day Kinfumu died, a nurse and a nun who cared for him fell ill. The nun was evacuated to another town, 70 miles to the West where she died -- but not until the contagion had spread to at least three of her fellow nuns. Two subsequently died. In Kikwit, the disease raged through the ranks of the hospital's staff. Inhabitants of the city began fleeing to neighboring villages. Some of the fugitives carried the deadly virus with them. Terrified health officials in Kikwit sent an urgent message to the World Health Organization. The Geneva-based group summoned expert help from around the globe: a team of experienced virus hunters composed of tropical-medicine specialists, virologists, and other researchers. They grabbed their lab equipment and their bubble-eye suits and clambered aboard transport planes headed for Kikwit.

Except for a handful of patients too sick to run away, the hospital was almost abandoned when the experts arrived. Supported by many others who were already there or soon to arrive, the response to the outbreak was headed by virologist Jean-Jacques Muyembe and epidemiologist David Heymann. Both went to work rapidly applying forceful methods to hamper and then stop the spread of Ebola infection.[9] They first identified patients who had traveled to the capital, Kinshasa, and isolated them. They began educating the community about the risk of infection and the need for proper containment. Finally came tactics for persuading the community to forego dangerous funeral rites: they must not congregate around or touch deceased family members and friends, not wash out a corpse's mouth, not wash the body, and not clip fingernails or hair. The DRC government tried to cordon off the city to prevent inhabitants from spreading the contagion across the countryside and into the sprawling slums of Kinshasa. The quarantine was only partly effective, as it had been years since there was a functioning government in DRC. The international doctors sent people with bullhorns through the streets pleading with residents to stay at home.

The next strategies were: 1) Rapidly identify and isolate those infected with Ebola virus; 2) Require health care workers to use protective clothing; 3) Institute health surveillance teams that followed locals contacted by Ebola-infected patients and monitor their temperatures twice a day for 3 weeks. Those with fever were isolated until disease was confirmed or excluded. Those testing positive for Ebola were hospitalized. 4) Educate individuals in the population area at risk on how to protect themselves and their families. Work by several international agencies, namely the Red Cross and the Red Crescent Societies, met with village elders and chiefs to distribute information tailored to local customs, that is, identify tribal remedies and funeral practices to avoid and prepare village leaders to advise members of their villages accordingly; 5) Provide protective gear for those transporting patients to hospitals for medical care and for those performing burial services.[9]

The identification of Ebola virus infection encountered endless difficulties. Specimens were collected and forwarded via the Belgian Embassy to the Institute of Tropical Medicine in Antwerp for evaluation. But the specimens could not be tested there for diagnosis of Ebola, because that institute no longer had the appropriate containment laboratory (BSL-4) for such studies. In Belgium, as elsewhere including the United States, short-term political considerations had reduced funding for surveillance as well as research for Ebola. The samples then traveled from Antwerp to the Centers for Disease

Control in Atlanta, Georgia, where tests were performed and identified those patients infected with Ebola virus. Locally around Kikwit, the road blockades enforced by DRC military were not effective at confining residents. Regardless of fever surveillance, fear drove both the sick and well villagers to avoid main roads, use forest paths to the Kikwit river, then travel further by boat.

Nevertheless, the restricted measures taken prevented the spread of Ebola infections to the large city of Kinshasa. The 1995 outbreak in Kikwit was limited to a recorded 316 Ebola-infected persons with 243 deaths, a mortality of 77%. This number is likely a low estimate of the disease spread and does not include those not identified who were ill and died in rural areas.

As we will see, the subsequent failure to contain the 2013-2016 Ebola outbreak in West Africa stemmed from a breakdown of several protocols that should have been followed. For example, in 2014 a quarantine failed at an urban slum in the large city of Monrovia, Liberia. That quarantine had no chance of success, because it was lifted just days after its declaration when armed members of the population clashed with the government forces.10 As a result, the infected residents and others mixed then moved freely in and out of the quarantined area. They avoided checkpoints and used bribery. Further, this was a more mobile population with better transportation (cars and motorcycles) and roads than those dwelling in Central Africa.

By this time, the Ebola virus had been characterized as belonging to the family of filoviruses, so-named for their long and thread-like shape that resembled filum, Latin for thread. Figure 1 displays an electron microscope photomicrograph of the virus emphasizing its length, up to 14,000 nm, varying 800 to 1200 nm, and its narrow diameter of only 80 nm. The seven genes comprising the viral genome total 19 Kb, which is large for a negative single-strand RNA virus, but small for most DNA viruses.

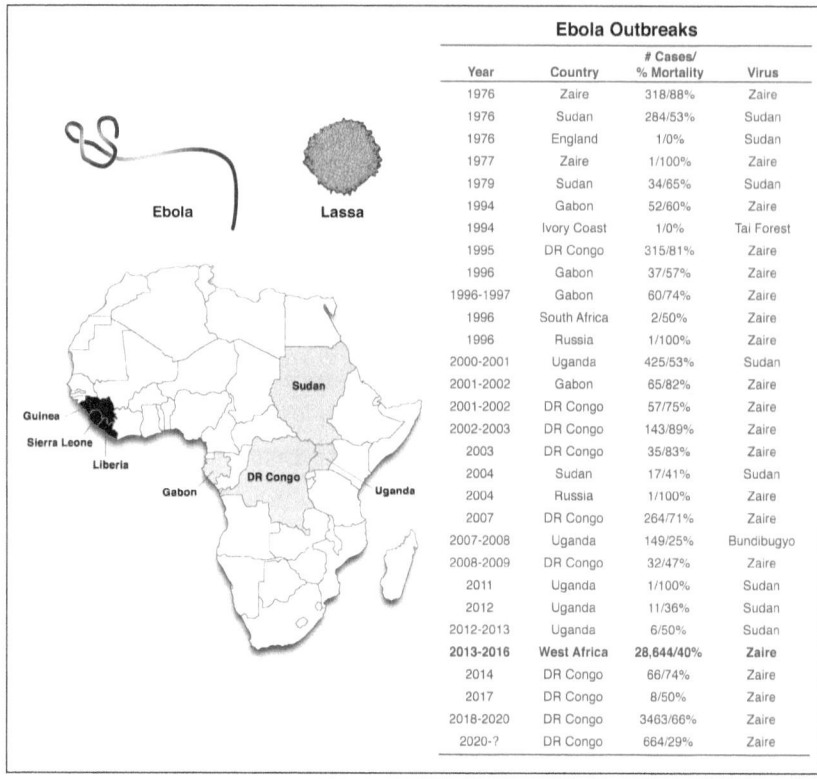

Ebola Outbreaks			
Year	Country	# Cases/ % Mortality	Virus
1976	Zaire	318/88%	Zaire
1976	Sudan	284/53%	Sudan
1976	England	1/0%	Sudan
1977	Zaire	1/100%	Zaire
1979	Sudan	34/65%	Sudan
1994	Gabon	52/60%	Zaire
1994	Ivory Coast	1/0%	Tai Forest
1995	DR Congo	315/81%	Zaire
1996	Gabon	37/57%	Zaire
1996-1997	Gabon	60/74%	Zaire
1996	South Africa	2/50%	Zaire
1996	Russia	1/100%	Zaire
2000-2001	Uganda	425/53%	Sudan
2001-2002	Gabon	65/82%	Zaire
2001-2002	DR Congo	57/75%	Zaire
2002-2003	DR Congo	143/89%	Zaire
2003	DR Congo	35/83%	Zaire
2004	Sudan	17/41%	Sudan
2004	Russia	1/100%	Zaire
2007	DR Congo	264/71%	Zaire
2007-2008	Uganda	149/25%	Bundibugyo
2008-2009	DR Congo	32/47%	Zaire
2011	Uganda	1/100%	Sudan
2012	Uganda	11/36%	Sudan
2012-2013	Uganda	6/50%	Sudan
2013-2016	**West Africa**	**28,644/40%**	**Zaire**
2014	DR Congo	66/74%	Zaire
2017	DR Congo	8/50%	Zaire
2018-2020	DR Congo	3463/66%	Zaire
2020-?	DR Congo	664/29%	Zaire

<u>Figure 1</u>. Left Panel: Upper displays electron micrograph drawing of Ebola and Lassa. Lower: map of Africa where Ebola broke out in Central Africa (gray) and outbreak in West Africa in black.

Right Panel: Chronologically lists all Ebola outbreaks as to year, location, number of cases and percent mortality, and Ebola strain implicated. The outbreak in West Africa is highlighted in bold black.

Despite advances in ascertaining the molecular biology of Ebola virus, the immune response in the human host to the virus, and its infectious nature, neither the biology nor pathogenesis is completely understood. Research is hampered, because Ebola is such a dangerous and severe human pathogen that it cannot be handled in a conventional laboratory but only in the highest-level containment facility known, a so-called Biosafety 4 laboratory (BSL-4). Scientific handlers had to be enclosed in specially designed space-like suits under positive pressure.

Recently in the 2018-2020 outbreak a number a number of air-conditioned cubicles to isolate Ebola patients became available. When used, health care workers did not wear the usual protective garments and could administer therapeutics and care for patients through portals outside of the cubicals. Additionally, virus outbreaks occurred intermittently then disappeared as an infectious agent only to reappear eventually (Figure 1).

Viruses contain either RNA or DNA and are, therefore, categorized as RNA or DNA viruses. Ebola as well as Lassa, to be described later, are the main viruses that produce hemorrhagic diseases in Africa, and both are RNA viruses. RNA viruses are the only organisms known to use RNA as their genetic material. They replicate their RNA genome in one of two unique ways. First, by either RNA-dependent RNA synthesis (Ebola, Lassa, and most RNA viruses [i.e., measles, influenza, poliomyelitis, etc.]), or second, by RNA-dependent DNA synthesis, so-called reverse transcription, followed by DNA replication and transcription (retroviruses like HIV).

Importantly, RNA replication is error prone, since this class of viruses does not have a strong proof-reading mechanism that corrects errors by removing wayward or mutated nucleic acids. The enzyme (polymerase) that catalyzes RNA replication has a minimal proof-reading activity. As a result, error-prone rates in RNA viruses are approximately 10,000 (1×10^4) times greater than those found in DNA viruses (i.e., herpesviruses, smallpox), whose proof-reading apparatus removes aberrant viral DNAs during DNA replication. Thus, the consequences for evolution, selection, and biology of RNA viruses are considerable. RNA virus populations never represent a homogeneous clone but instead embody a swarm of related RNA sequences clustered around a master sequence. This swarm is termed "quasispecies" and provides a fertile source of genetic variants that can respond to selective pressures such as infecting a resistant host. As a result, parts of the virus' genetic composition can change for its advantage. Thus, substitute amino acid(s) may lead to gain of function that results in increased virulence of the virus as seem by enhanced infectivity, replication, and spread. Thus, RNA viruses like Ebola can evolve up to one million times faster than DNA viruses and alter their established profile.

The high error rate of RNA viruses places a restriction on their genomic size, that is, the number of genes carried by the virus. Various RNA viruses carry from 4 to 13 genes; by comparison, DNA viruses (like herpesviruses or smallpox virus) carry hundreds of genes. DNA viruses, while requiring only a relatively few genes for their replication, carry a suitcase of many genes to provide the virus with a selective advantage. This suitcase contains accessory genes, not vital to the virus replication but important for enhancing the virus' survival and production of progeny. Hence, RNA viruses with far fewer genes must do as much as DNA viruses that contain a multitude of genes. RNA viruses accomplish that task in part by encoding proteins that perform multiple tasks. For RNA viruses, this enhanced diversity leads to numerous individual progeny and loss of many viruses from the swarm due to lethal virus mutation. The advantage for RNA viruses like Ebola and Lassa is a rapid evolutionary response.

Finally, RNA viruses are further divided into positive- and negative-strand varieties. Viruses with a positive-strand RNA deliver their genomic RNA directly to cells' machinery (ribosomes) to begin their infectious cycle. Positive-strand messenger RNA (mRNA) viruses are infectious and include those like poliomyelitis and Coxsackie. By contrast, Ebola and Lassa are negative-strand RNA viruses. Their RNA is not infectious. These viruses must begin their infectious cycle by transcribing (copying) viral mRNAs. This reaction is catalyzed by enzyme(s) carried into the hosts' cells by the infecting virus.

The natural reservoir of infection for Ebola virus is unclear.[11,12] Monkeys, other bush animals, and fruit bats can be infected by the virus and serve as intermediate hosts. Infected monkeys spread the disease to humans when they enter the human food chain or by blood contamination during butchering. Bats are believed to spread the disease by both their saliva, which then infects the fruit they suck/eat, parts of which are recovered and used in drinks consumed by humans, and by their use as a source of food.[3] Thus, man is an interloper who accidentally comes in contact with fluids or tissues from infected monkeys and bats. Once humans are infected, the virus replicates rapidly and is excreted in body fluids like tears, sweat from skin, blood, vomit, or diarrhea. It is the human-to-human spread of disease that causes epidemics.[3,5,13] Not until the fundamental public health approach of rapid diagnosis, quarantine, which prevents contact between sick humans and their healthy counterparts, and the rapid burials of the stricken dead is the spread of disease halted. To restrict disease spread, susceptible persons must be removed from all sources of infection.

In Central Africa, the migration of persons from village to village is limited by dense jungles, lack of easily accessible travel routes, and few vehicles for transport on land or water. Thus, outbreaks of disease usually remain within one village and do not necessarily penetrate surrounding communities. By experience in Central Africa, once Ebola appears in a village, locals often isolate sick persons to a single place so that person-to-person contact is avoided. Food and liquid are left outside the isolation hut or house, which is then destroyed by fire after all the infected person(s) have died.

In contrast, West Africa has more accessible paths, roads, and means of travel that facilitate human migration throughout one area and across/back-and-forth borders of several countries. Further, since only one single case and no major outbreaks or infection of multiple individuals with Ebola occurred in West Africa before the recent 2013-2016 epidemic, the experience of healthcare workers was limited, and the disease itself was not considered a top priority in this part of Africa. That single case of Ebola was located within the Ivory Coast (Cote d'Ivorie) in 1994. The cause was transmission of Ebola from an autopsy performed on a diseased chimpanzee found in the Taï Forest. The sequence identity between Ebola-Zaire of the Congo and the Taï-Ebola virus was only about 65%. Experience in West Africa and lack of public encounters or memory limited planning for what to do and how to monitor the local population if Ebola broke out in West Africa. Therefore, controls to limit person-to-person contact, discontinue hazardous tribal burial traditions, foster quarantines, and deal with the fear of viral spread were not yet sufficiently established in the susceptible population.

Ebola's Unanticipated
Arrival in West Africa

The Ebola epidemic of 2013-2016 duly arrived in Guinea, West Africa, at the remote village of Meliandou in the district of Guéckédou, which bordered two other West African countries, Liberia and Sierra Leone.[1] At that time, in December 2013, Meliandou was a rural forest community that farmed and hunted for its food supply to serve its occupants of just 31 huts. Chimpanzees and fruit bats were both known sources of meat for the village and both can harbor infectious Ebola virus.[2] How the Ebola-Zaire virus, which first appeared a thousand miles away (2,371 airline miles) in the Congo, in the heart of Central Africa in Yambuku 37 years earlier (1976),[3] now reared its head in Meliandou, West Africa, remains a mystery.

Emile Ouamouno, a 2-year-old boy, was known to have been exposed to and eaten both chimpanzee and fruit bat food. Villagers also reported a tall, scarred and hollow tree at the edge of Meliandou that housed a large colony of bats they called *lolibelo*. The tree was about 160 feet from the Ouamouno's hut and close to a small river used for washing. Local children, including Emile, frequently played in the hollow tree. Nearby, bats also hung under roofs of buildings.

In early December, Emile developed fever, vomiting, and passage of a black stool. Although his excretions were not examined for hemoglobin, a tarry or black stool is suspicious for oozing of blood or bleeding in the intestine. Four days later Emile was dead. From the onset of his disease on 2 December 2013, through 26 March 2014, 11 neighbors died in his village (9 deaths from 2 December 2013 to 8 February 2014; 2 deaths on 26 March 2014). First, Emile's mother died on 13 December, his 3-year-old sister became sick on the 25th of December and died on 29 December. His grandmother died 1 January 2014; a nurse became ill on 29 January and died 2 February 2014. Finally, a village midwife became sick, was taken to the hospital at Guéckédou on 25 January, and died on 2 February 2014.[4]

Soon, in nearby villages like Dandou Pombo and Dawa, and then in medical centers like the Guéckédou Hospital and other neighboring health care sites and hospitals, similar deaths followed, all victims of *Ebola's curse*. Dr. Kalissa N'Fansoumane of Guéckédou remarked …"we thought it a mysterious disease." For example, from the neighboring village of Dawa, the sister of Emile's grandmother and a friend, both attended the grandmother's funeral in Meliandou. They followed the local custom of touching and washing the dead person's body. Upon returning home to Dawa, both became ill in late January with fever, diarrhea, vomiting, and bleeding, and they died before the end of January 2014. Eight such deaths were recorded in Dawa from 26 January to 27 March 2014. As for the adjoining village of Dandou Pombo, there were six deaths from 11 February until 31 March 2014. The disease was introduced there by a midwife from the Meliandou village who became ill after being cared for by a family member at the village of Dandou Pombo. So on and on, the virus traveled from village to village to village. In the district Guéckédou Hospital, a health care worker passed the sickness on to others there, and those who became infected passed Ebola to the Macenta Hospital. Patients who died at Macenta Hospital had funerals in the village of Kissidougou. As a consequence of the funerals, five deaths followed on 26 March 2014, Ebola virus had been transported from Macenta to Kissidougou.[5]

After an unconceivable lag period of over three months, on 10 March, hospitals and public health services in Guéckédou and Macenta finally alerted the Ministry of Health in Guinea of their attack by an unknown "mysterious" fatal disease. Two days later, Doctors Without Borders (**Médecins Sans Frontières [MSF]**) were alerted about clusters of a mysterious disease characterized by high fever, diarrhea, vomiting, and an extreme fatality rate. Also in March the World Health Organization (WHO) was notified of the outbreak caused by an unknown pathogen that was devastating the region and rapidly spreading. The worrisome aftermath was that bureaucratic neglect had allowed a delay of over 100 days (109) after the first death occurred. Only on 23 March 2014 was WHO to declare that the viral disease in West Africa was caused by Ebola.[6]

An investigative team from the Guinea Ministry of Health reached the outbreak areas by 14 March; the MSF arrived on 18 March. Epidemiologic investigations were undertaken. Doctors Without Borders requested help to identify the etiologic agent responsible for the mysterious disease. Blood samples were collected and sent to the high-level BSL/4 containment laboratories in Lyon, France, and Hamburg, Germany. In those laboratories, RNA was extracted from 50 to 100 l of plasma (a teaspoon contains 500 l), diluted in RNA amplification reagent and searched for novel viral sequences that would be recognized as different from other infectious agents and markers of the patient. An additional 100 l of serum (blood fluid after removal of blood cells) was mixed with cultured cells to seek the expression and growth of a foreign agent. Cells used for this process were Vero E6, and supernatants from the cultures were repeatedly passed through the cells (process to amplify infectious agent). To identify the virus, antibody to several suspected infectious agents was applied in the hope of producing a reaction. Since the two most prevalent African hemorrhagic fever viruses are Lassa (common in that area of West Africa) and Ebola (except for one case in 1994 yet to appear in West Africa), these infectious agents were the major suspects. The results were unexpected and astonishing. The Pasteur group, led by Sylvain Baize, discovered that Ebola was involved in the outbreak and the Zaire strain was the one involved.[7] Of the blood samples collected from 20 patients, 15 were positive for Ebola virus. In virus recovered from culture and subjected to electron microscopy, 1 of 2 tested showed a portrait characteristic of Ebola (Figure 1).[7,8] None of these samples analyzed by any of the assays used was positive for Lassa fever virus or other suspected infectious agents (typhoid, malaria, yellow fever, etc.).[7] Thus, for the first time, Ebola virus infections of epidemic proportions were present and spreading in West Africa. The Pasteur group, in response to the French Ministry of Foreign Affairs, established a diagnostic laboratory in Macenta, Guinea. The report of Ebola in Guinea was rapidly placed on the internet on March 23, 2014. The data were observed by members of the Viral Hemorrhagic Consortium at the Broad Institute, Boston, and two participants of that group, Kristian Andersen and Stephen Gire. Andersen and Gire left Boston and arrived in Sierra Leone at the Kenema Government Hospital Lassa fever ward to set up a diagnostic polymerase chain reaction (PCR) assay for specific detection of Ebola. Although at this time there were no cases of Ebola in Sierra Leone, the investigators reasoned that in time, due to a close and open border with Guinea and the continuous exchange of individuals through both countries open borders, it would just be a matter of time when Ebola paid a visit. Unfortunately, this prediction came to fruition within a short time. The complete sequencing and bioinformatic data obtained from samples of Ebola virus variants circulating in infected patients in West Africa showed over 96%

(96.8%) identity to Ebola-Zaire strains from the Democratic Republic of the Congo in Central Africa.[9]

The epidemiologic survey assigned the outbreak index (first) case to Emile Ouamouno, the 2-year-old boy from the Guinea village of Meliandou (Figure 2).

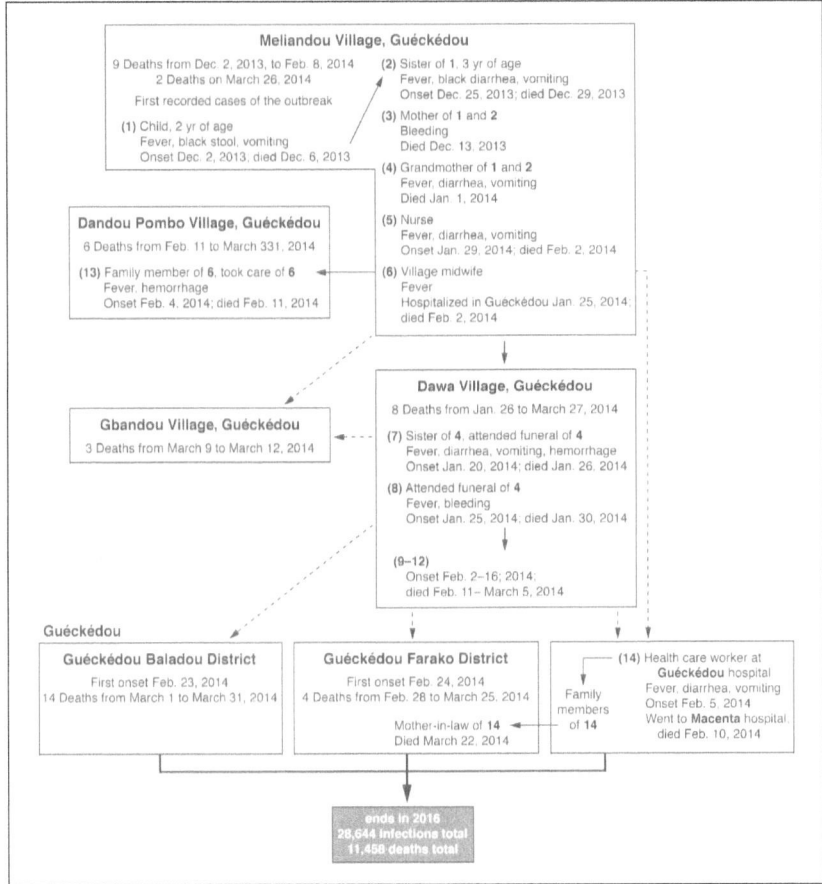

Figure 2. The index case (Emile Ouamouno) from the Guinea village of Meliandou believed responsible for the onset of 2013-2016 Ebola virus epidemic in West Africa and the initial spread of the infection.

Emile's diet was known to contain meat from animals (chimpanzee, fruit bats), previously established as reservoirs for Ebola virus. A background check noted that Emile played in a partly hollowed-out tree where bats resided. Epidemiologists learned that the hollow tree in question caught fire and burned in late March, a few months after Emile died, and ..."a rain of bats came out of the tree."

Researchers collected and tested bats in the area and showed they carried the Ebola-Zaire strain.[10] Other scientists at the Robert Koch Institute in Berlin, including ecologists, veterinarians, and anthropologists later surveyed wildlife forests near Meliandou.[11] They found no evidence of a die-off among larger animals such as monkeys, which can be susceptible to Ebola, and suggested that perhaps some other yet to be identified animal might be responsible for the viral transmission to man.[11] Fabien Leendertz, leading the study stated ..."We spent eight days in Meliandou. They told us that they regularly catch bats, like every other village in Guinea, Sierra Leone, and Liberia. The evidence is not 100%, and we can only say that this is the possible source of transmission. I would not say that the virus has emerged from central Africa. However, there are huge colonies of bats which regularly migrate. They can travel far in one night. I don't think an individual bat or colony migrated all the way from Congo or Gabon to West Africa. These big colonies are connected. There is a possibility for the virus to mix between colonies. They (the bats) share the same fruit. It is likely not to have even been one species of bat. The virus may jump from one species to another."[12] The team also collected samples of blood and tissue from captured bats, and the resulting data revealed they contained Ebola virus, suggesting that the reservoir host was most likely bats.

Like chimpanzees, bats carry the virus and could transmit Ebola via a soup made from bats considered a delicacy in Guinea. During the Ebola outbreak, Guinea banned the consumption and sale of bats for food in hope of preventing further spread of infection. Regardless, many natives in rural areas continued to hunt, procure, and eat bats and other bush meat.[11,12] This practice proved to be a continual difficulty for controlling the spread and transmission of disease. Also, failing to convince the population to stop cultural practices like touching and bathing sick persons and the dead enabled the high viral titers in skin, tears, and saliva to continue their deadly onslaught by passage to new susceptible individuals.[13,14]

Burials have been a prime source of spreading Ebola virus infection.13 Common religious rites of family and friends have created an overwhelming problem in containing the spread of the virus. In West Africa many cultural beliefs and religious rites after death includes washing, kissing, and touching the bodies of the deceased with bare hands.[13,14]

Certainly, the optimal safety procedure to protect the living from becoming infected with Ebola is for buriers to remove the dead body while wearing full protective gear, seal the body in a bag, drench the bag in bleach, and place it in a grave six-feet deep and fully covered. Unsafe burials played a substantial role in the spread of the virus. According to the WHO, "At least 20% of new Ebola infections occur during burials of deceased Ebola patients."[13,14] However, frequent push back and agitation between families and health workers interfered.[14] Sheku Bockaire, a Kenema Hospital health officer explained that ..."putting people in body bags creates a lot of suspicion in the minds of people; they think parts of the body are being cut, and that's why the body is not being allowed to be displayed."[15] One of the WHO's top Ebola experts, Pierre Formenty, recommended stronger cultural sensitivity. By building trust and respect between burial teams, bereaved families and religious groups, we are building trust and safety in the response itself. Introducing components such as inviting the family to be involved in digging the grave and offering options for dry ablution and shrouding will make a significant difference in curbing Ebola transmission."[13-15]

Death rituals in West Africa are rooted in a mixture of cultural and indigenous traditions as well as religious beliefs (predominantly Muslim and some Christian).[16] The rituals behind traditional funeral practices are strongly held. Burials are seen as necessary to put the deceased's spirit to rest so that the ancestor doesn't remain to haunt the living. Death rituals begin by preparing the home of the deceased for mourning. Mirrors and pictures of the dead individuals are removed. Although these are not items for spreading the virus, removing the deceased's bedding is, since virus is transferred in bodily fluids embedded in fabrics. Similarly, the rite of removing clothes from the deceased before wrapping the corpse in a sheet is a major problem, again because large amounts of infectious virus are found in sweat, tears, and bodily fluids of clothing from the deceased. Finally, according to customary ritual, the deceased must be buried correctly otherwise his/her spirit will haunt the living and cause harm. Such rituals and fears ingrained in many years of tradition and passed down through generations explain why families of deceased Ebola patients are both distraught and angered when told they cannot bury that person "correctly."[16] This situation worsened in Liberia, after communities ran out of proper burial sites, and the government ruled that bodies were to be cremated. As a result, many people avoided hospitals, attempted to remove family and friends from hospitals, and conducted secret burials. In several instances health care workers were bribed to hand bodies over to families.[17] Desperate to avoid force cremation of their loved ones, many families began paying private retrieval teams to help hide the infected bodies from the hospital. These private groups issued certificates from the Ministry of Health stating that the patient is free from Ebola and thus can be released back to the family; Prices of certificates range from $40 to $150. In addition, healthcare workers were being paid to produce fake death certificates making it difficult to track where bodies were buried. Those who are not able to hire these retrieval teams resorted to strikes and violence, causing workers to demand higher "risk" pay in fear of being attacked.[18]

Sierra Leone and Liberia share a border close to Meliandou and the Guéckédou district in Guinea where the first outbreak of Ebola occurred in West Africa (Figure 3).

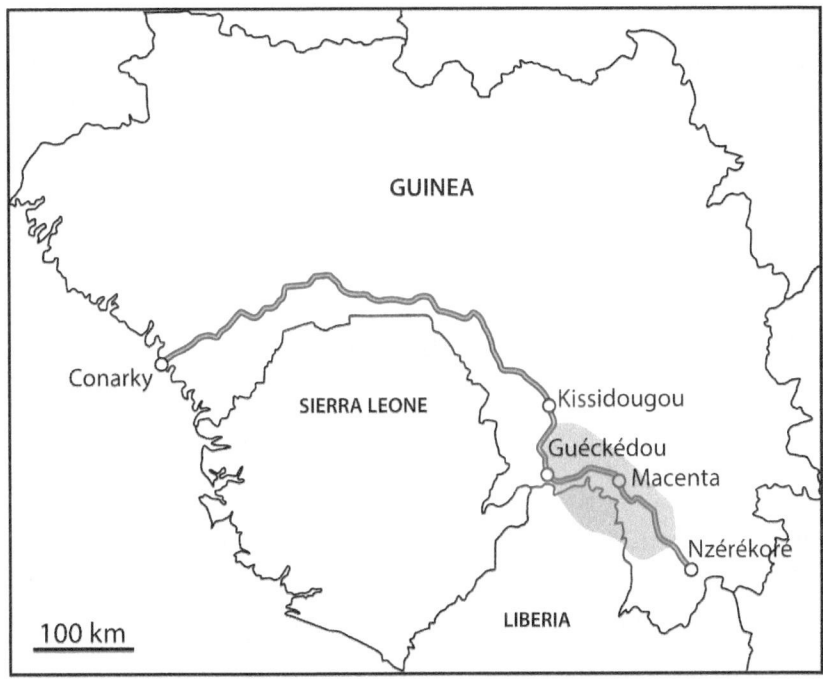

The first incidence of Ebola virus infection reached Sierra Leone on 24 May 2014. A young woman was admitted to the Kenema Government Hospital (KGH) after having a miscarriage.[19,20] Hospital staff workers were alerted and suspicious of Ebola infection due to its rapid spread, number of cases occurring in nearby Guinea, and the clinical presentation of the patient. A blood test using the PCR protocol set up earlier by Kristian Andersen and Stephen Gire confirmed that the young woman was positive for Ebola virus, and she was placed in an isolation medical unit. At that time there were 14 isolation beds available at KGH. Following her admission and treatment, no patients or staff at KGH contracted Ebola. The patient made a full recovery and was discharged. Afterward, health care workers and doctors at KGH began tracing back the source of her infection and its location. Their investigation determined that the patient had contracted the virus at the burial of a traditional native healer.[5,19,20] That healer was a female shaman and well-known for her mystical powers in and around the area of Kenema in Sierra Leone and bordering Guinea. Finda Nyuma's reputation not only included medicines she made from herbs in the forest, but also as people in and around her village area believed she communicated with the dead. Many came to her with messages to give to their dead family and friends. "They often found her beneath a bamboo palm, reading the future by throwing "jagay", small white cowrie shells."[20] The Ebola outbreak in Guinea relentlessly grew uncontrolled, patients from Guinea traveled to the healer in Sierra Leone in search of treatment. Eventually, the famous healer died from Ebola infection. First, Finda Nyuma's relatives, neighbors, and friends came to her room to say farewell and prepare her for her afterlife. It was believed that she would then become an ancestor (spirit) who, in exchange for tribute and respect, could intervene with spirits on their behalf. Later, hundreds of mourners from many villages traveled to congregate at her funeral and subsequent burial. There, the cultural practice of touching, washing, and lying on the body was again followed. As a result, 13 people at the funeral became directly infected. From these 13, the virus spread to over 300 other individuals resulting in as many as 365 deaths. Ebola was on the march to Sierra Leone. That march would result in Ebola-sickened victims fleeing to KGH which was approximately 63 miles from the healer's burial site in Koindu. The viral hemorrhagic isolation ward at KGH with only 14 beds for 14 patients, was soon to house as many as 80 Ebola virus-infected patients lying on floors and in halls. The hospital staff soon became overwhelmed, working close to 18 hours daily, and was to lose its head medical doctor Sheik Umar Khan, head nurse Mballu Fonnie, and nearly 50% of its staff.

Kenema Government Hospital: From Lassa to Ebola

The Kenema Government Hospital (KGH), located 186 miles from the Sierra Leone capital of Freetown, is a large public health facility in this Western African country. Interest in the city of Kenema and the population surge there correlated with the discovery of diamond mines and building of a railroad in the 1930s. Kenema, now a major trade center with a population of just under 200,000, is the third largest city in Sierra Leone, after Freetown and Bo, and is the largest city in the Western province. For many years, KGH has provided medical service to the city of Kenema and surrounding areas. Currently, the hospital has approximately 200 beds. During 2003, after the end of the civil war in Sierra Leone, KGH established an advanced clinical and research center to manage Lassa fever, the major virus-induced hemorrhagic fever that was and is endemic in this part of Africa. Initially, the Lassa virus treatment center run by the Viral Hemorrhagic Fever Consortium comprised physicians and health care workers from Sierra Leone as well as those from Tulane University Medical School in New Orleans, Louisiana.[1] The Sierra Leone Ministry of Health and Sanitation and the Viral Hemorrhagic Fever Consortium established a research program and also worked in tandem to provide diagnosis, surveillance, investigation of cases and tracking of contacts.[1] Since rodents are the natural vector for Lassa fever virus,[2-4] a plan for rodent control as well as community outreach and education followed. Funding for the Lassa research treatment program was/ is provided in part by the United States National Institutes of Health (NIH), Centers for Disease Control (CDC), World Health Organization (WHO), Merlin Group, and Ministry of Health and Sanitation of the Sierra Leone government. Although the early Lassa treatment center at KGH had only 14 beds, this facility came to play a pivotal role in treatment for victims of this major African hemorrhagic fever virus. Unexpectedly, KGH was also destined to become a crucial participant in the oncoming Ebola virus onslaught of 2014-2016.

Lassa virus was and continues to be the major cause of hemorrhagic fever in Western Africa, infecting roughly 400,000 to 500,000 individuals per year and yielding a death rate of 30,000 to 40,000.[2-4] Areas of prevalence for Lassa virus infection extend from Guinea in the West to Mali in the North to Nigeria in the East. The Eastern province of Sierra Leone has the distinction of harboring the highest incidence of Lassa virus-induced disease in the world. Infection from Lassa virus can occur all through the year but peaks in the rainy season, November to April. Typically, Lassa virus causes a persistent infection of rodents, and the human index case usually results from infection with virus shed by rodents in their urine or other excretions. During the rainy season rodents most often seek shelter inside village huts where contact with humans and stored foods is virtually unavoidable. In any one year, Lassa viruses infect and kill far more persons than the other major African hemorrhagic fever virus, Ebola. Ebola, since the time it was first described to the present, including the major 2013-2016 outbreak, has infected and killed fewer individuals in total than Lassa virus does in one year.[4,5] However, both Lassa and Ebola viruses cause devastating diseases with quite similar clinical features.[2,4]

So far, Lassa infection has affected primarily the West African population within Sierra Leone and Nigeria. In comparison, although the news concerning Ebola is well-justified, the hype is more a reflection of our time provided by the popular press and by books like Richard Preston's *The Hot Zone* that have sensationalized and overstated Ebola's impact.[6] In that context, the importance of Lassa virus infection is virtually forgotten or unrealistically minimized.

Because of the high incidence of Lassa viral infection in Kenema, a Lassa fever isolation ward that is a center of excellence in the treatment and clinical research of this disease was built at KGH. KGH also serves as a base for treatment of the many other infections that occur in the area from malaria, yellow fever, tuberculosis, to intestinal parasites as well as other medical issues.

In the early-1970s, Dr. Joseph McCormick of the Centers for Disease Control (CDC) set-up a field site at the Nixon Memorial Hospital in Segbwema,[7,8] which was an investigative and treatment site at Ranguma 62 miles away from Kenema. This field station was established to investigate a then mysterious hemorrhagic fever first recognized in 1969 that affected five health care workers.[8] The initial report of this infectious disease by John Frame and colleagues in 1970, described the events recorded below.[4]

"Ms. Laura Wine, a nurse working in the small mission hospital, Church of the Brethren, in Lassa, Nigeria, was in good health until about 12 January 1969, when she complained of a backache. On 20 January she reported a severe sore throat, but the physician who examined her found no signs to account for her discomfort. The next day, she complained that she could hardly swallow; she had several small ulcers in her throat and mouth, an oral temperature of 100°F, and bleeding from body orifices and hospital-induced needle puncture wounds. By 24 January she was suffering from sleepiness and some slurring of speech; late in the day she appeared increasingly drowsy. On 25 January she was flown to Bingham Memorial Hospital in Jos, Nigeria. She died on 26 January after several convulsions.

A 45-year-old staff nurse, Ms. Charlotte Shaw, at the Bingham Memorial Hospital in Jos, Nigeria, was on night call when Ms. Wine was admitted on 25 January 1969. Ms. Shaw had cut her finger earlier picking roses for another patient. As part of her nursing care, Ms. Shaw used a gauze dressing on that finger to clear secretions from the patient's mouth. Only afterward did she wash and apply antiseptic to the small cut on her finger. Nine days later Ms. Shaw had a chill with headache, severe back and leg pains and a mild sore throat, a clinical picture similar to that of Ms. Wine, who had died eight days earlier. Over the next few days, Ms. Shaw had chills with fever to 102°-103°F, headache and occasional nausea. Seven days after the onset of symptoms, a rash appeared on her face, neck and arms and spread to her trunk and thighs. The rash appeared to be petechiae (small hemorrhages), and blood was oozing from several areas of her body. Her temperature was 104.8°F. By 12 February her face was swollen; she had shortness of breath, a rapid, weak pulse… became cyanotic (bluish)…had a drop in blood pressure. Nurse Shaw died on the eleventh day of illness. Autopsy showed the presence of fluids in each pleural (chest) cavity and in the abdomen. Thus, like Ebola virus infection, once established in a human, the infection afflicting these two nurses, spread to other susceptible humans.

A 52-year-old nurse, Ms. Lily Pinneo, working at the same Nigerian hospital, Bingham Memorial, had nursed both these patients and had assisted in autopsy of the second patient. She collected blood and tissue samples. On 20 February she too developed a temperature of 100°F…followed two days later by weakness, headache, and nausea. After another three days, she had a sore throat and petechiae and was admitted to the hospital. Since this was the third case in progression, the physician decided to send the patient to the United States for diagnosis and treatment. She was flown to Lagos, Nigeria, where she lay for four days in an isolation shed, and then to New York attended by a missionary nurse...She was admitted to Columbia University Presbyterian Hospital (New York City)...and was placed in isolation with full precautions.

Pinneo continued to be acutely ill with a temperature of 101.2°F. The first night after admission, her temperature rose above 105°F...She became extremely weak during the next six days...Specimens from Ms. Pinneo were carried to the Rockefeller Foundation Arbovirus Laboratory at Yale University Medical School in New Haven, Connecticut, for study..."...the patient recovered strength slowly, became fever-free and was discharged from the hospital on the 3rd of May 1969."

One month later, an experienced and internationally known virologist, Dr. Jordi Cassals of the Yale University Arbovirus Research Laboratory, after working in New Haven with specimens from the patient, Ms. Pinneo, became ill and developed symptoms compatible with the acute mysterious virus infection.[4] During his slow convalescence, virus was isolated from his urine. The virus was studied and assigned the name Lassa, after the region in Nigeria where it was first isolated. A short time later, a technician from the Yale Arbovirus Laboratory, traveled to Pennsylvania to visit his family over the Thanksgiving holiday, became sick and died from Lassa virus infection. Consequently, the Yale Arbovirus Laboratory decided not to perform any more experiments with Lassa fever virus and shut down research and handling of this infectious agent. *The New York Times* and other publications reported the virus "too hot to handle."[4] With the presence of highly pathogenic infectious agents, the construction of novel isolation units for study of such agents were required and designed. Now, to safely protect scientists and allow work on these infectious agents, biosafety laboratory

(BSL)-4 units were constructed and opened. Several years later, with several BSL-4 laboratories available, such "hot viruses" as Lassa fever and Ebola could be safely handled. Fifteen BSL-4 laboratories are now operational or planned and located in various areas of the United States. The BSL-4 laboratory at the University of Texas Medical School, Galveston, is the one where the former Yale Arbovirus Laboratory unit relocated after leaving New Haven.

Lassa, like Ebola, is an RNA negative-strand virus. Unlike Ebola, Lassa belongs not to the filovirus family but is an arenavirus family member.[2] The Lassa virus genome is segmented into two sections, each with an RNA segment encoding two genes (total of four genes, two on each segment); its size is roughly 10.7 kilobases, and as viewed by electron microscopy, appears as polymorphic sand-like round particles (Figure 1). In contrast, Ebola is larger at 19 kb, is a non-segmented RNA virus, encodes seven proteins, and by electron microscopy is long, thin and worm-like (Figure 1). The host that carries Ebola in the wild is uncertain, possibly the fruit bat, whereas the reservoir that bears Lassa virus in nature is known to be a rodent. At least one way in which Ebola and Lassa are alike is that humans are unintentional intermediate hosts who initially become infected by exposure to a persistently infected animal. The virus is then passed from human-to-human as an end-stage infection, which if not cleared, kills the host. The disease following either infection is severe, since both viruses are among the most deadly infectious agents known to man. Frequently, either virus contaminates an unsuspecting or over-burdened hospital worker taking care of ill patients or disposing of the dead. The index case usually comes from a rural area.

As a response to the high concentration of Lassa fever infections in Sierra Leone, near Kenema, Joe McCormick and colleagues established the first CDC field station to treat and study these patients in the 1970s. However, a civil war in Sierra Leone in 1991 made this station too unsafe as a work area, and the unit was closed. With their activities in Sierra Leone disbanded, the CDC moved the unit to Guinea where their work continued.

The bloody civil war broke out in 1991 when a rebel army, the Revolutionary United Front (RUF) led by Foday Saybana Sankoh formed as an anti-government guerrilla warfare group and fought to overthrow the existing government of Joseph Momoh.[9] The RUF rebels began by attacking sites along the border of Liberia and Sierra Leone and quickly expanded to take over Eastern Sierra Leone. This guerrilla group gained prominence through murder, amputations, and child recruitment along with every form of fear and violence fostered by support from Charles Taylor's National Patriotic Front of Liberia (NPFL).[9] To finance the war the rebels took over the country's natural resources (diamonds). Thousands of children were kidnapped, drugged and forced to become soldiers in the rebel army.[10] Major instability followed throughout Sierra Leone with over half of the country's 4.6 million people murdered or displaced. Towns and government facilities were destroyed. The civil war lasted 11 years, disintegrated the economy of the area, and left over 50,000 persons dead. The overall result was loss of government authority, along with a displaced, homeless, starving, and sick population. The seeds of that disaster were to play an important role later in the 2013-2016 Ebola outbreak. Diseases such as Lassa fever continued unabated and added to the national crisis.

As a direct consequence of that civil war, one component of the Lassa virus research project in Sierra Leone was shifted to KGH. Dr. Aniru Conteh, a physician who had joined Joe McCormick and Sierra Leone's CDC team in 1979 and was trained in handling Lassa viruses, then moved to KGH where he became head of a Lassa investigation unit.[1] He and the team he had assembled wanted to continue their clinical and research work in Sierra Leone. Dr. Conteh devoted his life to treating patients with Lassa fever, becoming a leading world specialist in this infection.

KGH was left intact during the civil war and remained open. Despite the lack of security and resources, Dr. Conteh and his staff continued their work on Lassa fever. Over the 11 years of 1991-2002, the KGH staff treated thousands of patients, including the civilian native population, UN peacekeeping forces, and civil war fighters. Simultaneously, hundreds of individuals with Lassa fever were treated at the Lassa unit by Dr. Conteh. In March 2004, Dr. Conteh, while handling samples from a Lassa fever patient, sustained a needle stick, became infected with Lassa fever virus and died 18 days later. Sheik Umar Khan, then a recent graduate from the medical school in Freetown, was selected by the Sierra Leone government to succeed him as Director of the KGH Lassa unit.[1]

In 2004, the KGH Lassa unit established a partnership with Tulane University School of Medicine, New Orleans, Louisiana.[1] For some time, Tulane had been the principle partner with the Mano River Union Lassa Fever Network program, composed of WHO and ministries of Sierra Leone, Guinea, and Liberia. This diverse group of organizations strove to develop national and regional prevention and control strategies for Lassa fever in Africa, as well as performing laboratory research to better understand the pathogenesis of this hemorrhagic disease. Bob Garry, Professor of Microbiology at Tulane University Medical School, became the principle investigator (head) of the Viral Hemorrhagic Fever Consortium in 2003-2004 and remains in charge of building and maintaining this program to study Lassa fever virus infection. A Lassa fever isolation ward of 14 beds, the only such isolation ward in the world, was established at KGH and run by both Sheik Khan and a clinical physician from Tulane. As a consequence of the Ebola infection, the isolation ward was expanded to 42 beds. Health care workers were responsible for patient care, directing clinical research after approval by the appropriate institutional review committees, and training of other health care workers. The Lassa fever ward was and is physically separated from the rest of KGH and had its own staff of approximately 40. Anyone in Sierra Leone suspected of having Lassa fever was sent to KGH where medical care was/is free. Those with a confirmed diagnosis of Lassa fever were then admitted to the Lassa fever isolation ward, where regulations were strictly enforced. That is, medical and health care personnel were required to wear protective gowns, gloves, masks, and face shields. In place was a Lassa fever program that, in addition to providing hospital isolation and treatment, included a clinical research wing and fostered both Lassa virus awareness and ecology teams. The awareness team of five persons worked on outreach efforts including case investigations, surveillance, and public education. The ecology team of four trapped rodents, collected samples, and investigated contacts, their locations and their travel routes to and from areas suspected of contamination. On occasion, members of individual teams worked with/on another team. Clinical research was performed only after approval by institutional committees set-up by KGH, the Sierra Leone government, funding agencies such as National Institutes of Health (NIH), CDC, and participating American medical schools or institutions. A routine clinical Lassa laboratory was located on the grounds of KGH, and a separate BSL-2 suite was available for handling samples from patients with suspected Lassa fever. This BSL-2 laboratory enabled staff with expertise and the necessary equipment to identify Lassa virus. The research and BSL-2 program were overseen by Augustine Goba of Sierra Leone and Robert Garry from Tulane University School of Medicine. Goba, director of the KGH Lassa laboratory, diagnosed the first case of Ebola virus infection in Sierra Leone using PCR assay, and Garry was involved in the development of a rapid diagnostic test to detect Ebola.[11] Pardis Sabeti and colleagues from the Massachusetts Institute of Technology (MIT) Broad Institute and the Harvard University Medical School were brought in to sequence viral isolates and part of the human genome.[12] Although work with the whole infectious virus requires a BSL-4 facility, tests using individual viral proteins could and were done in a BSL-2 facility; as was handling of infectious blood in endemic African countries.

It was in this setting that the first Ebola-infected patient arrived at KGH in March 2014.[13,14] Rapidly, following the appearance of this virus-infected woman, first 10 to 20 then hundreds of sick successors appeared in March and June, all afflicted with a mysterious lethal infection soon diagnosed as Ebola. The research team knew that Lassa fever is spread on objects contaminated by infected rodents or by products contaminated with blood or tissues from infected patients and usually peaks in November through April, during the rainy season when rodents seek shelter in village homes. Now masses of ailing locals were arriving but not at the expected time when Lassa infections prevail. Soon the numbers of patients seeking medical help swamped KGH, changing the hospital's priority from Lassa virus to an Ebola treatment and clinical care center. Before 2014, Sierra Leone had no known case of Ebola infection, but in 2014 to mid-2015 there were over 8,000 and up to March 2016 over 14,100.[13,14] The outreach teams and surveillance programs available for the surrounding countryside soon became overwhelmed and inadequate. It was in this mix that Sheik Khan, his hospital staff, Bob Garry, Augustine Goba and his laboratory staff, and a young physician from Tulane, John Schieffelin, were to confront the rising tide and a continuous influx of sick and dying individuals infected with Ebola virus. Augustine Goba, for his work and dedication during the Ebola outbreak at the KGH Lassa unit was awarded a Presidential Citation from the Sierra Leone president, Bai Koroma..."...In recognition of his diligent and dedicated service in the fight against Ebola, especially as a viral hemorrhagic laboratory scientist who diagnosed the first Ebola case in Sierra Leone and led the Ebola testing nationally until other Ebola diagnostic laboratories were established."[15] John Schieffelin, as a result of his experience, published a definitive report on the clinical presentation of Ebola infection[16] ...Sheik Umar Khan's experience was far worse.[1,17]

He died after contracting the disease from infected patients. His deputy, Donald Grant, a Sierra Leone physician, then replaced him.

For Schieffelin and his colleagues, the unexpectedly tremendous influx of Ebola patients provided a large trove of data to characterize clinical features of the disease.[16] First, he was able to confirm the observations of others regarding the clinical presentation of fever as the most common symptom (89% of patients had fever), weakness (66%), dizziness (60%), diarrhea (51%), abdominal pain (40%), vomiting (34%), with only 1% presenting with bleeding. Among the novel findings were variability of how individuals responded to the virus with some having mild cases and others going downhill quickly. These findings correlated with the Ebola viral load carried in their blood. Of those having 100,000 (1×10^5) copies of virus per millimeter of blood, 67% survived, but only 6% survived a viral content of 10,000,000 (1×10^7) copies/ml. Determining what impact the innate immune response had (i.e., patients' production of type 1 interferon, other cytokines and chemokines, macrophages, natural killer cells, etc.) or the effect of adaptive immunity (virus-specific T cell responses, antibodies) was undertaken by my laboratory working at KGH from 2015-2016. Analysis of the immune system, genetic sequencing of Ebola virus and of patients studied were /are the subjects of active investigation in my laboratory (M.B.A. Oldstone) and those of Garry, Sabeti, Anderson and the KGH Lassa unit.[18] The results are vital to inform those who will generate efficient and effective vaccines and adoptive antiviral therapies.

Another issue raised from investigation of the Ebola outbreak is the possibility of one human being a super viral spreader.[19,20] That is, were exceptionally large groups of susceptible humans infected by one especially virulent individual or source (a "super spreader") or did many much smaller groups become infected by similar contact with multiple infected individuals? How/if the answer to these questions apply and whether the answer might relate to differences in total virus content carried by an infected host are unknown. After amino acid sequencing of several Ebola virus genomes, we do know that the cause is probably *not* genetic variations (mutations) in the virus.[20,21]

With the increased numbers of Ebola infected individuals in Guinea and the first cases from areas just a three- to four-hour drive away, Garry departed New Orleans and quickly returned to KGH sensing an absolute need to be physically present to direct and participate in educating the staff and obtaining protective equipment for health care personnel before the Ebola infection reached Sierra Leone in large numbers and control of the infection was lost. As Garry later related, despite his frequent pleas…"…unfortunately we did not get much help from the international community and the outbreak really spun out of control". "From the emergence of Ebola in 2013 to May 23, 2014, there were officially 258 diagnosed or probable cases of Ebola viral-induced disease, all in Guinea or Liberia. The WHO was only days from announcing that the outbreak ended when Augustine Goba diagnosed the first Ebola case in Sierra Leone. Subsequent investigations revealed that the outbreak had not been confined to Guinea and Liberia, instead the official numbers under-estimated the true number of cases of Ebola virus."[13,14,22]

Despite the growing numbers, some believed that the Ebola outbreak would burn-out in as soon as weeks to months. In an interview on National Public Radio in the United States on June 18, Robert Garry disagreed and recounted the deaths in the vicinity of Daru, but his warning was depicted as needlessly alarming. Doctors Without Borders was another group that appealed for more international assistance at this time but was likewise labeled alarmist. Because the internet is unreliable in that area of West Africa, Garry made frequent trips to KGH in Sierra Leone alternated with travel to the U.S. in attempts to raise funds to combat Ebola, Garry remarked…"…In June 2014, [I] was one of the few saying this outbreak could take a spin for the worse and spin out of control. Unfortunately, international response was way too slow. International effort in public health (was needed) to stop disease."[11] The Viral Hemorrhagic Fever Consortium headed and run by Garry was targeted on research to understand the pathogenesis of Lassa fever infection and was not a public health consortium. Actual public health solutions to contend with Ebola required many boots on the ground for diagnosis, isolation, education, large scale case tracking, and disposal of the dead.

As Garry related ..."...some help came but not enough." "...like a train speeding down the track. People running after it, but not enough people to actually get them to stop it..." "This outbreak is so much more massive than anything that anybody has ever been confronted with before. The prior outbreaks -- you can look them all up (see Figure 1) -- have all been in middle Africa. And they've been in small villages that were very isolated. It's much easier to get those patients isolated. Middle Africa doesn't have the road structure, doesn't have the population density, that is there in West Africa. People move around a lot; the roads are good in West Africa. Remember, there are diamonds there, and that means that there is a very interesting geography and lots of valuable minerals...So mining companies have built a lot of good roads, and there are a lot of people moving around. So that is a recipe for the virus to be able to spread quickly."[11]

At KGH, a staggering number of sick individuals kept coming. There, Sheik Khan and other doctors from Sierra Leone, Tulane, and elsewhere were on the front line. The case load of KGH increased beyond its capacity. Nurses from other parts of KGH were recruited...but personal protective equipment was in short supply. By the middle of July 2014, several members of the nursing staff had been infected with Ebola virus. One of the nurses who became infected was pregnant. Four nurses, including the head nurse of the KGH Lassa ward, Mbalu Fonnie, who worked with the Lassa fever program for over 25 years, attempted to save the life of their nursing colleague by inducing a still-birth delivery, a procedure that offers a chance of survival for the pregnant mother.[26] Despite their best efforts though, the pregnant nurse died; then each of the four treating nurses became infected with Ebola virus. All four died, including nurse Fonnie. John Schieffelin, an Assistant Professor of clinical medicine and pediatrics, having finished his residency training at the Louisiana State University Health Science Center in New Orleans and Tulane University in 2009, went to join the Viral Hemorrhagic Fever Consortium to pursue his interest in clinical infectious disease and antibody responses. He was sent through a WHO program. At the KGH prior to the Ebola outbreak, he had profiled Lassa virus-infected patients as part of a WHO program that sent him there. Therefore, Schieffelin was present when Ebola broke out and during the massive influx of Ebola virus infected individuals. After joining Sheik Khan they worked together in the designated Lassa virus infection ward. At times, as many as 80 to 90 patients occupied that facility with only 14 beds . Those care providers were stretched much past their capacity, working 16- to 18-hour shifts. Schieffelin, as a result, saw a multitude of Ebola-infected patients and was able to provide one of the best and most thorough descriptions of their clinical manifestations and outcomes.[16] The result was sadly different for Sheik Khan. Khan became infected with Ebola, becoming one of its victims. This loss of health care workers had a devastating effect on their colleagues and co-workers. As stated by Garry ...".."...These people are my colleagues and my friends. I've been working with them for 10 years. It's devastating to have lost these very valuable colleagues and people that I care about. That's irreplaceable. Dr. Sheik Umar Khan, who you may have read about, caught Ebola. He was a person I worked with for 10 years. His legacy will be -- he will be missed. We'll carry on. We'll move forward. But this is a person who it is impossible to replace. Nurse Mbalu Fonnie, we've been working with her for 10 years, but she's been doing Lassa fever research for 30 years. You can't just replace that kind of experience and know-how and find somebody who knows these things overnight. So, yeah, it's going to be a rebuilding process when this is over."[11]

"You just do what you can. Obviously, the people who are working with the patients and are the ones on the front line of the treatment and are trying to give care to these people who are infected with Ebola are at the greatest risk. In the laboratory environment, that's a more controlled environment. We can feel more secure in there. But there's always a chance that a mistake is made...and so, yeah, these are considerations. This is high-risk work."[11]

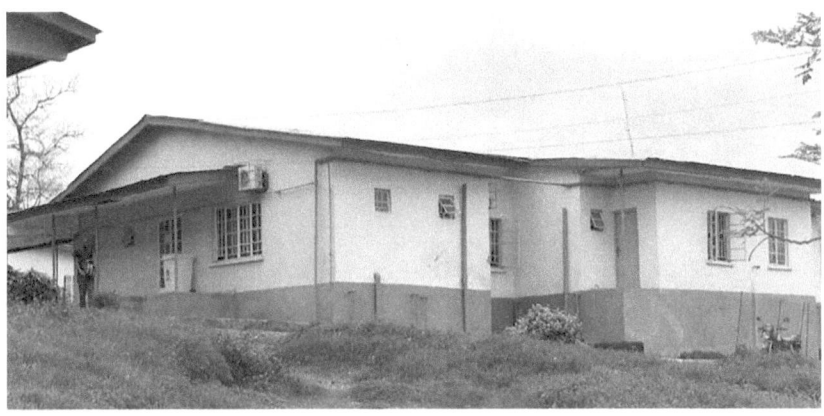

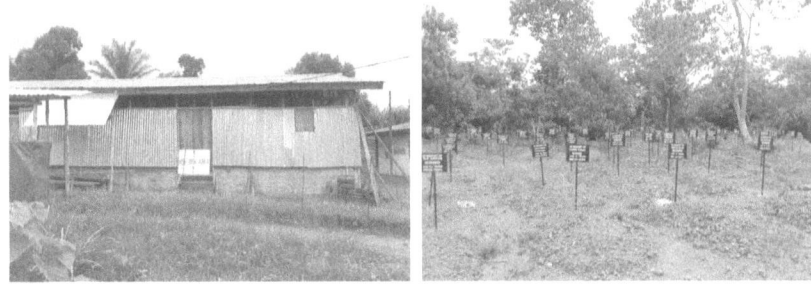

Figure 4.

Top: KGH.

Lower left: Holding area were individuals were assessed as to whether they were infected with Ebola and were to be admitted to KGH or whether they were not infected and were discharged.

Lower right: Displays the burial area located outside the hospital. Photographs taken by and a gift from Kristen Anderson, The Scripps Research Institute

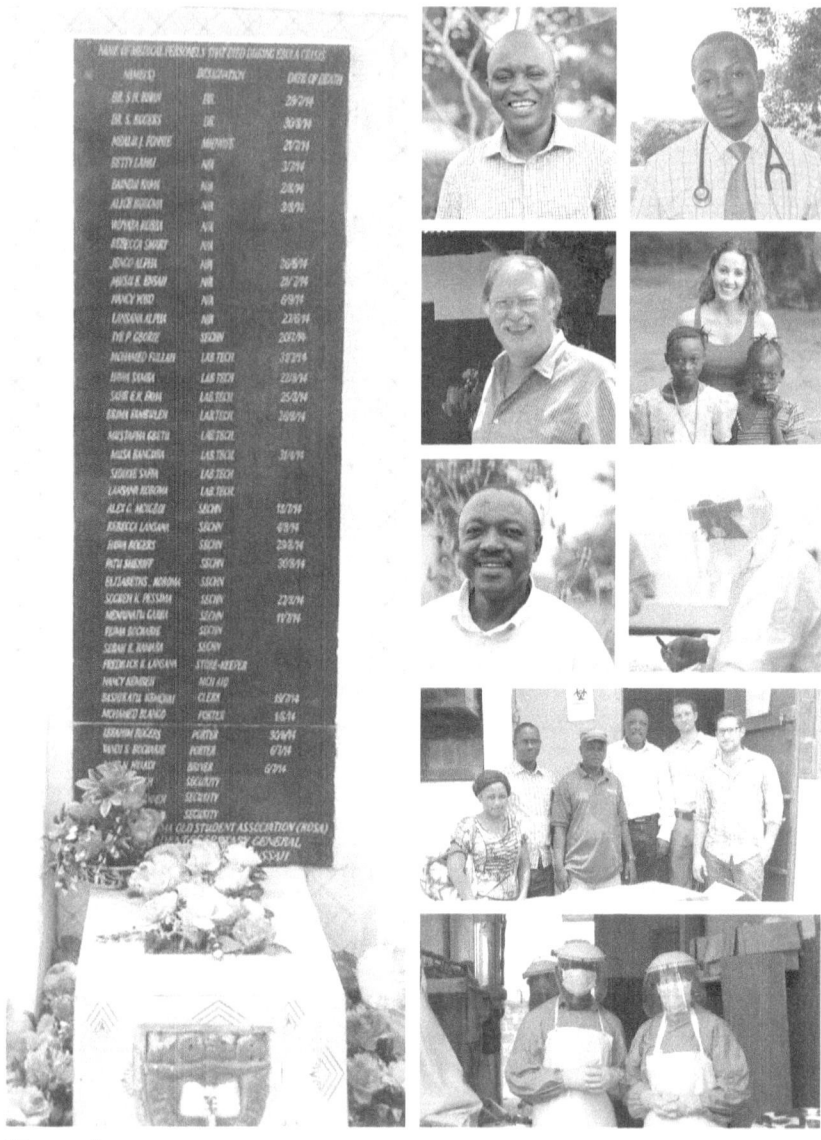

Figure 5.

Left panel: Shows the monument dedicated to the health care workers of KGH who lost their lives while engaged in the fight against Ebola.

Right panel: Shows several of the prominent workers at KGH who played a role in the Ebola outbreak in Kenema 2014-2015. From top to bottom, left to right: Sheik Umar Khan, David Grant (1st row); Bob Garry,

Pardis Sabeti (2nd row); Augustine Goba, and a protected worker in the laboratory (3rd row); health care workers and MIT geneticists, from the right are Drs. Gire and Andersen, next to lab head Goba (4th row). Photographs taken by and a gift from Kristen Anderson, The Scripps Research Institute

Sheik Humar Khan: Leading the Fight Against Ebola in Sierra Leone at Kenema Government Hospital

On 29 July 2014, in his 39th year of life, Dr. Sheik Humar Khan died from Ebola virus infection and was buried on the grounds of Kenema Government Hospital. His colleague Dr. Pardis Sabeti with Bob Katsiaficas composed this song for him and other health workers who succumbed to the deadly Ebola virus while serving their patients in Sierra Leone.

One Truth

Verse 3
A lifetime that we write
We laugh
We cry

We pray
We are love

we dream
we scream
we strive

our hunger will never die
I'm here in this fight, always
A lifetime for one for one truth
That I'm alive, And so are you
We are here, We are the proof
Yeah

A lifetime for one for one truth x 3

As a remarkable, humanitarian gesture, Sheik Humar Khan and the KGH team came to the fight against Ebola with boundless energy and passion. Among them was a background of many years' expertise in the diagnosis, care, and treatment of the major African hemorrhagic disease of West Africa, Lassa fever virus, a plague that annually infected the Sierra Leone population.[1,2] Then, in 2014, a wholly unanticipated outbreak of Ebola virus in Sierra Leone quickly swamped KGH turning its Lassa fever ward into an Ebola center. Better prepared than most hospitals with a staff trained to wear protective garments and use their anti-viral armamentarium to fight Lassa, they easily and quickly adjusted to Ebola. Thus, they came to wage a strong and competent fight against Ebola infection with experience and expertise gained from many years of exposure to Lassa. With the massive influx of cases, Sheik Khan's team expanded to over 40 persons including scientists, physicians, and medical care workers from Kenema, Sierra Leone, Tulane, Harvard, MIT, others from West Africa, USA, Europe, and Asia (Figure 5). Efforts were led primarily by Khan, Americans from

Tulane like Robert Garry, followed by John Schieffelin, as well as Pardis Sabeti and her crew from Harvard and the MIT Broad Institute. Donald Grant was recruited by the Sierra Leone government to replace Sheik Khan after his death and handle his responsibilities. While Khan, Grant, and Schieffelin, with head nurse Mballu Fonnie organized and provided medical services, Garry along with Augustine Goba, managed the diagnostic and research laboratory. In addition, Garry collected patients' blood samples to be analyzed for understanding their immune (antibody) responses; that is, were these responses fighting the infection or not? From these blood samples, they also obtained RNA to test the Ebola virus' genetic pattern for changes and mutations. Some samples were then sent to Pardis Sabeti, a trained physician and geneticist at the center for genomics, who was instrumental in studying infectious diseases. Further, Garry and colleagues collected and purified blood cells [leukocytes] from survivors of Ebola virus infection and sent these samples to my laboratory in La Jolla, California, to assay for CD8 and CD4 Ebola virus-specific T cells. Later in 2015-2019 Brian Sullivan and several postdoctoral fellows from my laboratory travelled to KGH to study immune responses to both Ebola and Lassa fever viruses in those individuals who survived the disease.[3,4] In addition a few individuals acutely infected with Lassa fever virus were also analyzed. Funded by the World Bank and the NIH, Sabeti and her colleagues originally set up the instrumentation, bioinformatic programs, and personnel to analyze the genomics of LASV in Nigeria and at KGH, but with the tidal wave of Ebola cases, they also took on the genomic study of Ebola.

Additionally, and importantly, Garry shuttled multiple times between Africa and the US, attempting to raise funds to purchase protective equipment for the health providers, supplies for patient care, and resources to keep the KGH isolation ward functional (Figure 4). His main concern, though, was to alert the WHO and Americans at large of the current Ebola disaster's ever enlarging scale and its coming threat.

When Ebola killed Dr. Sheik Khan in July of 2014, he had treated over 100 patients bearing that infection. He was working shifts of 16-18 hours/day administering to their overwhelming sickness, despite the lack of supplies. Overworked and exhausted, he became an easy target for the virulent Ebola virus. To honor his work, sacrifice, and his good life and premature death, Khan was recognized by Sierra Leone's President Ernest Bai Koroma and termed a "National Hero" of the country.[5] On the grounds of Kenema Government Hospital a memorial monument was dedicated to him and to those at KGH who lost their lives in the fight against Ebola (Figure 5). The LASV ward being rebuilt to a 42 bed unit was named after him. As a tribute from the United States, the American Society for Microbiology established the Sheik Khan Lecture and Prize at its annual national meeting. The first such named lecture was presented by Heinz Feldmann of the NIH, National Institute of Allergy and Infectious Diseases, Rocky Mountain Laboratories located in Hamilton, Montana. Feldmann, who directs the BSL-4 laboratory there, had been working with Ebola viruses and continues to do so. He knew and interacted with Sheik Khan. Sheik Khan was posthumously awarded the 2015 Ed Nowakowski Senior Memorial Clinical Virology Award from the Pan American Society for Clinical Virology, which was accepted in his absence by his brother, Sahid Khan.

Sheik Khan was born in 1975 into a large family of nine brothers and sisters. The parents and some brothers and sisters live in Lungi, a town not far from Freetown. Sheik Khan in his youth dreamed of a medical career. Growing up he frequently addressed himself as "doctor" in the presence of family and friends. His dream became a reality when he was accepted to, schooled at, and graduated from the University of Sierra Leone College of Medicine and Allied Health Sciences. During that time, Khan became deeply interested in Africa's infectious diseases, particularly LASV, Ebola, malaria, tuberculosis, HIV, and AIDS.

After graduating from medical school, Khan took a one-year internship with focus on tropical medicine and infectious diseases. He was recruited as a Medical Officer by the Directorate of Disease Prevention and Control Ministry of Health and Sanitation, in Sierra Leone. After two years in this position and with the death of Dr. Aniru Conteh, the hospital's former Director, Khan applied for and was accepted for the open position as head of the KGH Lassa fever program.[6,7] That few applicants wanted the position was no surprise. Work with a dangerous pathogen like Lassa fever virus requiring hours in the BSL facility was not popular. Further, many Sierra Leone physicians were hesitant to move away from the academic centers where they trained and leave better economic opportunities. But Khan saw the bigger picture of KGH as worthy and a worthwhile prospect for a successful future. His involvement as a consultant for the Mano River Union Lassa Fever Network brought him into a special scientific relationship with Robert Garry and the Tulane group and Pardis Sabeti and the Genomic Center at Harvard/MIT Broad Institute.[7] As its Chief at the KGH LASV facility, Khan ran the LASV program for almost a decade. His knowledge and professional experience in viral hemorrhagic fever diseases attracted the attention of the United Nations. He was contacted by the United Nations Mission in Sierra Leone (UNAMSIL) as a physician consultant for Lassa fever in Sierra Leone. From 2005 to 2010, Khan working at KGH was the physician in charge of HIV and AIDS regional services as well as LASV. From 2010 to 2013, Khan temporarily left his post at KGH to complete an internal medicine residency at the Korle Bu Teaching Hospital in Accra, Ghana. With the outbreak of Ebola, though, he completed his studies and returned to his position as physician in charge of the Lassa fever program. Nevertheless, Khan, like many, feared the lethal virus. He stated ..."I am afraid for my life. I may say…health workers are prone to the disease because we are the first port of call for someone who is sickened by disease." Khan's courage, work ethics, personality and charge to fight Ebola inspired not only the KGH staff but many of the international colleagues, collaborators, and friends he knew. His predecessor, Dr. Conteh, had pricked himself with a needle contaminated with blood from a woman who had LASV, and he died 12 days later of LASV infection. At the time of Khan's appointment, he was all of 30 years of age and hardly tested in administration, running a service or handling large influxes of LASV infected persons. However, in retrospect, he turned out to be an excellent choice to fill the position. He learned quickly and earned the respect of the KGH Lassa medical care staff, Robert Garry and the Tulane group, as well as Pardis Sabeti and the Harvard/MIT Broad Institute participants; they and others who interacted with him voiced their high regard while later mourning his death.

With the Ebola outbreak, 14 beds in the KGH Lassa isolation ward were rapidly filled with sick and dying patients as were adjacent areas on the floors, halls, and outside grounds. The beds in the KGH Lassa ward were "cholera beds" - that is a mattress covered with plastic but punctured with a hole in the center. A bucket was placed under the hole to catch the diarrhea output. As the numbers of Ebola patients increased and Khan's stress magnified, he spoke for himself and his coworkers who were justified in their fear of dying from early and continual exposure to their sickened charges.

His family in Lungi were concerned and they asked him to consider leaving KGH and no longer risk his life. Khan's sister said ..."I told him not to go there" but he said..."If I refuse to treat them, who would treat me?" As the Ebola virus rampaged through West Africa, the Lassa containment unit at KGH became overwhelmed and filled by Ebola virus infected patients -- their number exceeding the available health staff, services, and beds. Khan became emotionally and physically depleted. Still, he stood bravely by his post when the outbreak occurred and continued, endlessly providing treatment. Not only was he in charge of leading the hospital, he also treated hundreds of patients himself. Meanwhile, he trained senior doctors and medical staff on precautionary measures as well as how to assist and treat patients. He was constantly on the phone with government officials to aid in coordinating control efforts and to raise needed funds.

Alex Moigboi, who worked in the hospital with Khan, was the first of the health care staff to contract Ebola. He died soon afterward. Then head nurse, Mballu Fonnie, became infected with Ebola. Fonnie, who had worked at the KGH Lassa ward since it first opened in the 1990s, died. Two other nurses, Fatima Kamara and Veronica Tucker, became infected. Many staff members at KGH became terrified, deserted the hospital/ ward and their work, never to return. However, Khan remained in the Ebola ward with less and less support and fewer and fewer supplies. The health care system was collapsing under the strain of Ebola. Elsewhere, other international medical groups were stretched thin. One such group, Doctors Without Borders, was barely coping with Ebola virus infected patients in several health care units including Kailahun, a town about 65 miles from KGH.

Khan talked regularly with Pardis Sabeti -- ..."we are all alone here," he told her. In addition to Bob Garry, Pardis and her colleagues were working hard to rush supplies and people to KGH. She told Khan ..."the most important thing is your safety." "Please take care of yourself." "People and help are coming." But it was not to be enough or in time. Khan told Pardis ..."I have to do everything I can to help these people." Khan was commanding and leading a battlefield charge, although many troops under his command were dead, dying, or fleeing.

In May 2014 the first patient with Ebola virus infection was seen, diagnosed and treated at KGH, but about four months later, on 18th July, Khan did not feel well. He had a blood test taken on the 21st July with results that confirmed he was infected with Ebola virus.[8] Because of the likely psychological impact, he did not want his remaining staff to see him develop the symptoms and signs of Ebola, thus further compromising their already low morale. So, Khan arranged for transportation to take him to Kailahun, the Ebola care and treatment center run by Doctors Without Borders.

At the Kailahun health center, as elsewhere, therapy was limited to patient care and fluid replacement. There were no proven pharmaceutical drugs available to directly treat the infection. However, the Kailahun Ebola care center did possess a potential but untested medical therapy, a cocktail of antibodies called ZMapp. Antibodies are proteins synthesized by specialized lymphoid cells in response to stimulation by a specific antigen, in this case antigen(s) (proteins) of the Ebola virus. By virtue of the antibody's two binding parts, it can attach to the specific viral antigen that elicited it, inciting a series of events that neutralize or block the virus from which the antibody was derived.[9] Antibodies may also attach and crosslink the virus, thereby lowering the numbers of virus particles present.[9] ZMapp was still an experimental antibody preparation and not yet tested in humans. During the two years between this 2013-2016 outbreak and the 2018-2020 outbreak in DRC, human subject approvals by appropriate African, NIH, WHO, Doctors Without Borders and pharmaceutical manufacturer committees to administer ZMapp to ill Ebola virus infected patients were obtained. Enough ZMapp and three other approved anti-viral drugs were then administered during the 2018-2020 Ebola viral outbreak. The results of that clinical trial and whether ZMapp was an effective therapy for humans is presented in Chapter 10. However, three months before Khan became ill, ZMapp had been given to monkeys infected with a lethal challenge of Ebola virus and fully protected them from developing the fatal disease. That protection saved the animals' lives even when the antibodies were given when the monkeys were ill, five days after receiving Ebola.[10]

It had been observed that humans previously infected with Ebola but survived resisted reinfection when exposed again to the virus. Also, although controversial, several reports insisted that blood (serum or plasma) taken from those previously infected and immune to the virus might be helpful as a lifesaving therapy for patients sick with Ebola. Theoretically, such blood could contain antibodies to Ebola and then administered as a so-called adoptive (transfer of antibody) immune therapy. The difficulty in knowing if protection from adoptively transferred antibodies was protective was because since not all Ebola infected patients die, it was not clear if those that survive after receiving adoptive immune therapy would have survived without the antibody therapy. Further, not all Ebola-infected persons given the antibody transfer survive. Nevertheless, with a ruthless disease and limited therapeutic options, the use of antibody transfer was the rationale for Mapp Biopharmaceutical Inc. in San Diego, in collaboration with the Public Health Agency of Canada's National Microbiology Laboratory in Winnipeg, Canada, to manufacture the ZMapp product. To do so, they isolated antibodies to Ebola from antibody-producing cells of individuals surviving Ebola infection or from mice immunized with Ebola virus. Such antibodies were then manipulated genetically to produce a strongly neutralizing product to be used as a therapeutic reagent. To enhance the amount of antibody made the investigators used tobacco plants from a biotech Kentucky firm, Kentucky Bio-Processing. By inserting genes for antibody production into these tobacco plants, a therapeutic compound was produced that could potentially treat patients infected with Ebola virus, and eventually yield large quantities of that compound to be used to treat the epidemic. However, before use for humans, the therapeutic ZMapp would have to first go through animal studies to show potency and then clinical trials in humans to show safety. ZMapp was shown to be effective against Ebola virus in tissue culture and in animal experiments.[10] However, its toxicity or therapeutic potential was unknown and untested in humans. Also, insufficient data were available to know how the ZMapp reagent would hold up in a less than optimal environment. The ZMapp stored at the Doctors Without Borders center in Kailahun would be a test of the compound's survival properties in an environment where electrical power often failed, and the climate was very hot.

The government of Sierra Leone regarded Khan's deepening sickness as a national crisis and sent out international pleas for any drug or therapy that might help him. A series of international conference calls were made to officials from WHO, CDC, NIH, U.S. Army Medical Research Institute of Infectious Diseases, Public Health Agency of Canada, ZMapp, and Doctors Without Borders where treatment for Sheik Khan was debated. In the end, the decision not to treat Sheik Khan was made on July 25th by Doctors Without Borders. Khan was not informed of the availability of ZMapp and he died four days later on July 29th. Of course, it was not known if ZMapp would work and whether it was toxic. This posed an ethical problem for treating West Africans because of the risks involved and past treatments of Africans.[11] Although one might argue, and we would, that Sheik Khan should have been told about ZMapp and given the option of receiving the therapy.

On July 31st there was a funeral for Sheik Khan in Kenema at KGH.[12] In attendance were over 500 people including the Sierra Leone governing health ministers, health care workers, and scientists who knew and worked with him. Residents of the town who joined them included many he had cared for. Sheik Khan was buried on KGH grounds, which were named for him. Before the Ebola outbreak, Sheik Khan had been scheduled to take a few months sabbatical with Pardis Sabeti in Boston to learn more genetics. Instead, he was buried on the grounds of KGH.[12]

ZMapp: The Ethics
of Decision Making

As thousands in West Africa and surrounding areas were infected with Ebola virus, and Sheik Khan lay infected and dying, Robert Garry's message to him was "we're working on vaccines and medicines for Ebola - the solutions are coming." Pardis Sabeti pleaded "take care of yourself, help is on the way." But neither vaccines nor pharmaceuticals were available as yet for use in the field resulting in Khan's and over 11,000 other deaths. Such treatments awaited the 2018-2020 outbreak in Central Africa (see Figure 1). Chapter 10 details the success and failures of such therapies. For Khan and others sickened in the 2013-2016 Ebola outbreak the only reliable therapy was fluids to replace dehydration and offset circulatory collapse resulting from fever and diarrhea. Accelerated studies to find pharmacologic remedies to treat infected individuals and the development of vaccines to prevent new Ebola outbreaks were under way in several industrial countries but had progressed no further than the developmental stage, testing in animals, or anticipated preclinical trials in humans.

The formulation of treatments for human viral diseases consists of two quite different approaches. The first is research at the molecular and cellular level to define the virus' life cycle in its quest to produce progeny virus and then screen for pharmacologic drugs that block reproductive stages of virus's life cycle. To gain knowledge of what self-components the virus requires to allow its survival and production of progeny while interacting with the host, both private and public libraries of known chemicals or synthesized compounds are searched. The goal is to identify molecules with the ability to block viral replication. Such assays require a robust readout and automation involving robotics to screen virtually millions of test molecules before identifying just a few (1-4%) that show promise. Any molecule identified requires, first, confirmation and, then, analysis that it is not itself toxic. Thereafter, chemists' study and modify its structure to optimize the therapeutic index, that is, the relative safety of a dose or treatment as opposed to its potentially harmful effect.

Achieving the maximal advantage for an eventual therapeutic product requires vigorous chemical and biological testing to evaluate the stability, half-life, and best route of delivery -- either oral, intravenous, subcutaneous, etc. Armed with this knowledge, the developers' next steps of discovery are to determine the pharmacologic molecule's effectiveness, usually first in cell cultures and then in animal models. For testing Ebola virus, animal models can include genetically modified mice, guinea pigs, or subhuman primates.

In the course of this search, hundreds of thousands of molecules are often screened before a therapeutic "hit" is uncovered. Unfortunately, and frequently, the molecule or compound identified is disqualified because of its toxicity, insolubility, or delivery problems. Chemists then work to alter the structure of the selected compound to overcome such difficulties.

The time involved can be and is usually long and the financial cost great. Nevertheless, this approach has achieved amazing success over the last few years. Examples are discoveries of drugs that changed HIV/AIDS infection from a near certain lethal event (mortality >90%) to a 1% or less death rate for HIV patients who are medicated daily.[1] However, these drugs are expensive and not always available in some countries. Similarly, the antiviral therapy recently discovered for chronic hepatitis C virus now cures over 95% of such patients instead of the lifetime persistent infection their predecessors suffered.[2] Additionally, the risk of developing liver cancer and requiring a liver transplant is greatly diminished. Although anti-hepatis C virus (HCV) therapy is initially expensive, compared to the former long-term hospitalization, likely transplant surgery or cancer treatment, the long-term cost is modest, and the value is great for patients as well as for the health care system.

In view of the successful outcomes with antiviral therapies, finding one or more molecules to combat ongoing Ebola infection seemed possible. An announcement had appeared that the small molecule, GS-5734, an adenosine analogue with antiviral activity, protected 100% of rhesus monkeys three days after initiation of a lethal Ebola infection.[3] The virus tested was the Makona variant of Ebola, the virus isolated during the outbreak in Sierra Leone during 2014. Of further interest was the drug's effectiveness against other filoviruses (Marburg), arenaviruses (LASV), and coronaviruses (SARS). Despite its promise, though, this therapy still required testing for safety and then clinical trials in humans. The issues of large-scale manufacturing and pharmacokinetics still needed resolution to determine whether a drug, if produced, would be available for the next Ebola outbreak. It was not yet available for Sheik Khan.

The second approach in the development of treatments for human viral diseases is harnessing the host's immune response most often by developing an effective vaccine. The immune system has evolved to enable the host to resist invasion by organisms like, in this case, Ebola virus. Proteins in Ebola that trigger an immune response are called antigens (immunogens).

A host's immune response to antigens can travel down two very different pathways. The most common and satisfactory one provides protection, controls the infection by either preventing it totally or lessening (attenuating) its effects and induces a protective immune response. Such a response can provide long-term protection from Ebola virus so that a repeated infection does not cause disease -- sort of one and done. To mimic that scenario, a vaccine is created to prime the immune response by programming it to recognize and then rapidly resist the Ebola infection in an individual who later becomes exposed to Ebola. Vaccines developed against viruses like measles, mumps, small-pox, yellow fever, poliomyelitis, etc., have changed the human and medical landscapes in that they succeeded in reducing the morbidity and mortality of human viral diseases.[2] This success stands as one of the greatest of public health advancements. For example, smallpox alone in the twentieth century killed an estimated 300 million individuals, about three-fold more than all the wars of the that century, including World Wars I and II. Vaccination eliminated smallpox so that, in the twenty-first century, not one case has emerged.[2] Similarly, if one is infected by and survives an Ebola infection, that person is immune to re-infection. Indeed, during the 2013-2016 Ebola outbreak, such "naturally immune" individuals, because of their resistance to re-infection by Ebola, often worked to provide care and trans-port patients.

How does the immune response evade or control viral in-fection? The immune system must discriminate between for-eign antigens, such as viral proteins, that are not found in humans (non-self) and those antigens that are self (your own proteins found in your cells and tissues). Cross-reactivity of a persons' immune response to the virus with the individual's own "self-proteins" can lead to an autoimmune (anti-self) response -- a response to *self*-components, and autoimmune diseases like lupus, multiple sclerosis, diabetes, or thyroiditis.[4]

After an initial exposure to viral infection, the so-called

acute phase, a race is on between the virus, which is replicating rapidly, and the host's immune system, which functions first to limit the amount of virus made and second to clear the virus from the host. At stake is whether the virus can or cannot successfully replicate and the infected person lives or dies. To combat the virus, the host mobilizes and uses many weapons, that is, both the immunologically specific and nonspecific responses. The nonspecific factors are all early combatants against the virus and the cells it infects. Included in this group are natural killer lymphoid cells, phagocytic macrophages -- large cells that ingest or eat viruses -- and proteins in the blood called complement factors that are capable of interacting with viruses and also destroying virus-infected cells. Important is the innate immune system that provides the initial defense against pathogens and primes the subsequent adoptive (T cell and antibody) immune response. The major players in the innate immune response are toll-like receptors, which recognize particular microbial patterns, and type 1 interferons (IFNs). Again, there are conflicting reports of whether IFNs are suppressed or exaggerated. Nevertheless, these innate systems are mutually complementary and are involved in developing the ensuing adoptive immune response. Type 1 IFNs upregulate molecules on cells that present major histocompatibility complex (MHC) molecules, molecules that code for self. MHC molecules are essential for optimal interaction with T cells. Following a virus infection or vaccination, antigen-presenting cells (called dendritic cells) present segments of viral proteins (peptides) that become located within MHC molecules to naïve T cells, an action termed "priming." By this means virus-specific T cells are generated and expanded numerically. These T cells are made in the infected host to specifically control the virus infection. Thus, the major combatants against viruses are antibodies and T lymphocytes, both of which mount the host immune response to Ebola, although the relative contribution of each is not completely clear. However, in this battle, within 10 to 14 days after infection, either the replicating viruses or the host's immune response will emerge as the winner. If the immune response wins, viruses are vanquished, and the host survives with enduring immunity to that virus. However, if the immune response is overcome, the Ebola virus infection ends in the host's death or in a small subset of individuals fingerprints of Ebola that can be found months later.[5,6]

What is the cellular (T cell) virus-specific immune response? The component parts are CD8+ and CD4+ T cells. The T stands for thymus-derived and CD8+ or CD4+ indicates a specific molecule present on the cells' surface used to identify the cell. The thymus is a two-lobed gland of the lymphoid system located over the heart and under the breastbone. Lymphocytes formed in the bone marrow (hemopoietic stem cells) migrate to and enter the thymus where they are educated (mature) and are then selected to become either CD8+ or CD4+ T cells. CD8+ T cells function as surveillance and killer cells, which accounts for their name "cytotoxic T lymphocytes" (CTLs). They travel along the highways of blood vessels and wander among tissues throughout the body seeking cells that are foreign (not like self), because they express viral proteins. CTLs then recognize, attack, and kill such cells. By this strategy they eliminate the factories making viruses. CD8+ T cells also release soluble factors like IFN-g and tumor necrosis factor-alpha (TNF-a) that also have antiviral effects but do so without killing the virus-infected cell. CD4+ T cells predominantly serve a different role. They release soluble materials (proteins) that help or induce bone marrow-derived (non-thymic-educated) B lymphocytes to differentiate and make antibodies. CD4+ T cells release soluble factors (cytokines) that also participate in clearing a virus infection and uncommonly CD4+ T cells may also kill virally infected cells.

In contrast to reacting against cells, antibodies react primarily with viruses in the body fluids and are, therefore, most effective in preventing the virus from entering a permissive cell to avert infection or by limiting the spread of virus through the blood or in cerebrospinal fluids, fluids that bathe the brain and spinal cord. By this means, antibodies decrease a host's content of virus and diminish infectivity. Antibodies lower the numbers of viruses thereby allowing CTLs to work more efficiently. Antibodies along with effector molecules like complement can kill virus-infected cells. However, this mechanism is relatively inefficient compared to CTL killing of virus-infected cells. Although over 10,000 or more viral antigens must be present on the surface of a virus-infected cell to achieve lysis by antibody, less than 10 viral antigens expressed on a cell and restricted by MHC are all that are needed for a CD8 T cell to do the job. Thus, during infection, the eradication of virus-infected cells is the primary job of CTLs, whereas antibody's main task is to first prevent infection and second if some infection occurs then curtail the spread of virus in body fluids.

Antibodies are made by differentiated B lymphocytes named plasmacytes. Once activated such cells can pump out 100 million antiviral antibody molecules per hour.

Antibodies latch onto and neutralize viruses by one of several mechanisms: 1) antibodies can coat or block the outer spike protein of the virus that is required to attach to the cell and begin its entry into the cell. By this means antibodies can prevent infection. This is a major action of vaccination. 2) Antibodies can aggregate or clump viruses so that the net number of infectious particles is reduced. 3) With the assistance of complement, antibodies can lyse (disintegrate) viruses, and 4) antibodies can react with viral antigens on the outer membrane of the infected cells to limit the manufacturing or transcription of virus molecules inside the cells, thereby restricting the amount of virus made. Each antibody molecule generated acts on a specific antigen or target molecule of the virus.

When a host is initially exposed to an infecting virus or to a vaccine containing viral antigens, antibodies specific for that virus as well as CTLs are generated. The CTL response is initiated on the first day of infection, expands over 100,000 to 1,000,000 times by doubling roughly every twelve hours with peak expansion seven to eight days after exposure. Thereafter, the quantity of these cells contracts and is maintained at 1 to 2 percent of the total generated: these become immune memory cells. Immune memory T cells are rapidly stimulated and accelerated to respond if the same or cross-reactive infection occurs. Antibodies that neutralize the virus peak after the CTL response often by 4 to 6 months after the virus infection has been terminated. According to Robert Garry who with his colleagues have worked on the antibody response, enough titers of neutralizing antibodies to Ebola virus are not detected until 4 months and peak by one year after the beginning of the infection. Antibodies that bind to the virus (virus-antibody immune complexes) are detected during the first two weeks following infection. Free [non-bound] antibodies are often weakly detectable during the acute phase of infection. The number of free neutralizing antibodies then rises, and they linger for years. Thus, in most virus infections, CTLs are the major players in purging virus and terminating the infection. Recently my laboratory identified the major virus components needed to generate a vigorous CTL response obtained from a population that survived the 2013-2016 Ebola infection in West Africa.[7] The inclusion of virus protein component(s) so-recognized by CTLs along with the virus glycoprotein to generate neutralizing antibody is likely to provide a most effective vaccine to protect against Ebola virus infection. Such a designed vaccine would mimic the successful immune response in previously infected individuals that cleared the virus and terminated the acute infection. Out data indicated that a vaccine containing the virus's outer glycoprotein coat or its components that block or limit virus entry into cells as well as virus molecules from inside the virion [nucleoprotein] was required to best generate a vigorous antibody and CD8 and CD4 T cell response.[7]

During an acute onset of a viral infection, the mechanics

of obtaining sufficient virus-specific CD8 T cells in humans to transfer into an MHC-matched individual is barely doable, even for study in a sophisticated clinical research center at an optimal hospital setting in the West. This task is not feasible during an Ebola infection in Africa. Yet, the transfer of convalescent plasma (plasma is blood from which red cells, have been removed) harvested from Ebola-immune donors into acutely ill Ebola patients is possible.[8] Such "immune" plasma (plasma containing antibodies to Ebola) can be placed in storage and thus remain available. The million dollar question is -- does this protocol work and, if so, of therapeutic value. For such transfers, blood is harvested in heparinized tubes to prevent clotting. T cells, red blood cells, macrophages, etc., are removed by centrifugation, and the resultant plasma is injected intravenously into the infected patient. In clinical trials with 84 patients of various ages acutely infected with Ebola virus, 200 to 250 ml of test inoculum was tested. This plasma was harvested from previously infected Ebola patients who survived the disease.[8] Unfortunately, though, the survival rate of these patients did not improve significantly over that of the controls who were not so inoculated. However, the study was flawed in that neutralizing antibodies to Ebola were not quantitated or adjusted in the transferred plasma. Thus, it is unclear whether the failure to treat Ebola successfully was real, or perhaps due to low concentrations of neutralizing antibodies in the plasma that was used. In other studies potent neutralizing antibodies against Ebola were isolated from B cell clones of individuals (immune) who recovered from Ebola infection.[9-11] One such antibody, mAb114, given only once, protected 3 of 3 macaques even when administered as late as 5 days into the Ebola infection cycle.[11] The one macaque given no neutralizing antibody died at day 10 post-infection with 10^8 logs of virus. Similarly, potent neutralizing antibodies were isolated from a survivor of the 2014 Ebola outbreak and 77% of the 349 monoclonal antibodies isolated neutralized Ebola indicating that a broad diversity of

B cell clones target sites on the glycoproteins of Ebola being generated during infection.[9,10] Impetus to develop this strategy further came from these results with Ebola and other studies in which monoclonal antibody provided protection against a hemorrhagic arenavirus infection of Argentina, Junin tested in A guinea pig model[12], and for anti-HIV-1 antibodies in a monkey model.[13]

An important consideration underlying the proposed development of a vaccine was the observed protection from Ebola virus infection in humans who survived the initial infection when re-exposed to Ebola. Such observations provided the scientific rationale and the logic for financial investment by government agencies like the National Institutes of Health (NIH) and charitable foundations to obtain an effective vaccine against Ebola. Less attention comes from most large pharmaceutical companies because from a commercial standpoint, even if successful, the vaccine would be used in an, as yet non-industrial (still third world) country; therefore, the market for a vaccine would be smaller and less profitable than in industrialized Western countries. Because of its high lethality, specialized facilities are essential for handling and testing Ebola. So far, insufficient data are available about the early events in humans of infectious process of Ebola infection; many acutely infected individuals are in poor physical condition, and handling the virus requires a high security laboratory.

Recently, soon after becoming infected with Ebola virus, 4 survivors were air transported from West Africa to Emory University School of Medicine.[14] The blood profiles of these post-acute subjects were analyzed at Emory and the CDC in selective BSL-4 facilities. Surprisingly, the individuals displayed exceptionally strong anti-Ebola T and B cell responses.[14] These observations were the opposite of early reports that T and B Ebola virus specific responses were suppressed. The cause of this difference could be temporal, that is, the timing of blood sample collection, the advanced methodology used or perhaps the survivor population studied. Analysis of specific anti-Ebola T and B cell responses during the early acute phase of disease is currently limited and conclusion unresolved. However, new and better facilities in West Africa, especially at Sierra Leone and KGH, as well as recent NIH support to identify and map T cell epitopes (regions on the virus as it comes to the surface of infected host cells) and funds to support virologists and immunologists from both Sierra Leone and the United States.[7] The importance is in identifying the arms of the host immune response against Ebola virus and in discovering the essential viral proteins to constitute a vaccine that provides optimal immunity and protection, thereby preventing infection and/or purging the virus.[7,14]

This background brings us back to the advancing death of Sheik Umar Khan from Ebola virus infection, the controversy about using ZMapp for his treatment and the ethics of administering an untested drug to severely ill persons. ZMapp was a cocktail of monoclonal antibodies, the first to be suggested two years earlier as a potential transfer antibody therapy for Ebola.[15] ZMapp, created through international cooperation, showed promising results in primates but had not been tested on or approved for human usage. The majority of research to develop ZMapp was funded by the National Institutes of Health and Public Health Agency of Canada. When the Ebola outbreak began, the question of its use was raised, although it had not yet been deemed safe or effective for treating humans. Tests with monkeys infected with Ebola had shown a protective effect when they were given ZMapp at 3-5 days after infection.[15] Could ZMapp have a similarly protective effect in humans? Also, ZMapp had been produced in tobacco plants, a procedure used to expand its production. Would there be an issue of sensitivity to tobacco antigens for humans in therapy provided intravenously?

"The evidence presented suggests that ZMapp offers the best option of the experimental therapies currently in development for treating Ebola virus infected patients. We hope that initial safety tests in humans will be undertaken soon" Gary P. Kobinger of the Canadian Public Health Agency's National Laboratory for Zoonotic Diseases and Special Pathogens stated.

As Sheik Khan lay dying in the Doctors Without Borders Care Center in Kailahun, and the debate of whether or not to treat him with ZMapp was raging, over 480 miles to the Northwest in Monrovia, Liberia, at Samaritan's Purse ELWA Hospital, another crisis was unfolding. Samaritan's Purse, a Christian Relief Ministry, was coming to grips with the fact that two of its health care workers involved in treating Ebola patients, Kent Brantly, a 33-year-old physician, and Nancy Writebol, a healthcare worker and missionary, showed clinical symptoms and signs of Ebola. The infection was confirmed by blood test. A hospital administrator for Samaritan's Purse, Lance Plyler, knew there were experimental drugs being developed elsewhere to combat Ebola. Losing no time, he contacted a CDC official stationed in Monrovia to obtain names and places in the United States to seek the necessary therapeutics. Meanwhile, the infected and quarantined Kent Brantly was surfing the net with his laptop computer for a potential and possible therapy for Ebola. Brantly came across the report in *Nature*[15] that ZMapp, a cocktail of antibodies to neutralize Ebola, saved monkeys challenged with a lethal dose of Ebola even when they were several days into their illness. However, ZMapp had been tested only in cultured cells or animals and not yet been shown to be harmless or effective in humans. Nevertheless, Brantly selected ZMapp as his choice. Was the material available? Lance Plyler contacted Gary Kobinger in Canada who was involved in the creation and testing of ZMapp. Plyler requested that the drug be sent to Samaritan's Purse Hospital for its immediate use. Kobinger informed Plyler that the nearest supply of the drug was only 480 miles away from the ELWA facility at the Doctors without Borders Kailahun Care Facility, where Khan was near death. Concerning Khan, the debate continued whether or not he should receive ZMapp. Plyler requested the drug and arranged for a helicopter to take ZMapp from the Doctors Without Borders Care Center to Monrovia.

The issue was the limited number of ZMapp treatments available, only five doses existed in all of Africa and who should be selected to receive it. ZMapp had been sent to West Africa to the Doctors Without Borders Care Center in Kailahun primarily to determine how the drug would hold up in the African environment of heat and electrical power failures. The plan was to then return the drug to Canada and re-evaluate its antiviral efficacy: was it stable; was there a loss in potency? Although a promising anti-Ebola therapeutic, ZMapp had not attracted robust funds for its development. In a CBS News interview, Dr. Jeffrey D. Turner, President and CEO of Defyrus, a private life sciences biodefense company that collaborated with public government public health agencies and military partners in the UK and Canada, stated "The challenge that many people don't appreciate is that our plans were to scale up this drug for 2015 and even then, small amounts for clinical trials. What has really happened with this outbreak is it's caught us in a position where we didn't have enough ZMapp available because no one would have bought it."

ZMapp was produced in a specific type of biologically-engineered, genetically modified tobacco plant, *Nicotiana benthamiana,* grown at Kentucky BioProcessing in Owensboro, Kentucky. The genes encoding the monoclonal antibodies made elsewhere were inserted in these plants and the plants then produced large quantities of the antibody. However, the manufacturing procedure takes several weeks. Production was comparatively inexpensive, since as many as 100 million doses of antibody could be made for $36 million. In addition to Kentucky BioProcessing, the biopharmaceutical companies involved in the development of ZMapp included San Diego-based Mapp Biopharmaceutical and Texas-based Caliber Biotherapeutics.

After Sheik Khan's infection with Ebola was diagnosed at Kenema Government Hospital, he asked for a transfer to the Doctors Without Borders Clinical Center in Kailahun to avoid further demoralizing his hospital staff. By chance, Kailahan was the site where ZMapp was stored. The question being debated by the doctors at that time was, should ZMapp be used for humans and, if so, in whom? How would these individuals be selected? It was into this setting that the severely ill Sheik Khan's name entered the debate. Initially and under pressure from the Sierra Leone government to do something for Sheik Khan, already recognized as a national hero in that country, the physicians treating Khan and others involved were presented with an ethical and philosophical dilemma. What if the patient died as a result of an allergic reaction to ZMapp? ZMapp had not undergone clinical trials for safety and efficacy in humans. What if the treatment failed? Many believed that Khan should receive ZMapp because, in all of West Africa, he was the leading and best known figure involved in the war on Ebola. However, other decision makers were hesitant. Also, the fact that Khan was African brought attention to the recent uproar that Westerners were subjecting Africans to a potential lethal therapy.[16]

After a heated argument, the authorities in charge decided against giving ZMapp to Khan. That decision would be unpopular and not in line with the general requests for help advocated by Khan's government and specific requests of his colleagues. Garry and Sabeti applied pressure that he should receive the therapy. Khan's blood had already generated antibodies to the virus, indicating that his own immune system was beginning to work to combat the viral infection. However, as discussed above, early reports that the virus could suppress the immune system remained under reassessment. There was also concern that the drug might affect his immune response. Khan was denied the ZMapp therapy but not told of its potential benefit or availability. Representatives of Doctors Without Borders said he wasn't consulted because it would be unethical to inform him of the potential drug that was not available to him. One of Khan's close friends and fellow researcher, Dr. Daniel Bausch, strongly disagreed, "Dr. Khan is the ideal person to make an informed decision, and I feel strongly that he should have been asked if he wanted it or not…that's one area where, frankly, I am critical." Nevertheless, shortly after being denied the drug, Khan died.

The next day, despite the same concerns that prevented ZMapp treatment for the dying Khan, other infected individuals, received ZMapp. The treatment that might have saved Khan's life was, instead, transported to Samaritan's Purse ELWA Hospital in Liberia and administered to two Ebola-infected health workers from the United States. This act created a strongly emotional response from the local population and the international community. Giving ZMapp to two Westerners who survived and not to Khan, an African who died, was highly controversial. Since not all those infected with Ebola die (mortality for the 2014-2016 outbreak was 40%), possibly the two Westerners would have survived without ZMapp. After all, many did. If Sheik Khan had been given ZMapp and died, would Africans be convinced he was used as a guinea pig to be tested with an experimental/unproved therapy without either formal local approval or approval by Western scientific and government committees? The two American recipients of ZMapp, Kent Brantly and Nancy Writebol, were members of Samaritan's Purse, the Christian Missionary in Liberia. A source from the NIH stated that someone from the CDC contacted Samaritan's Purse and that an NIH scientist later informed them of the drug. However, no one knew if the drug would work or if the ultimate recovery of those taking the ZMapp was due to the drug. After receiving ZMapp, Kent Brantly showed remarkable clinical improvement, although, in contrast, after receiving the drug Nancy Writebol's condition worsened. However, both Brantly and Writebol survived, but may have recovered without the ZMapp -- one does not know. The indisputable fact is that Sheik Khan died without receiving ZMapp when, with its possible/ potential therapeutic effect, he might have lived.

Many of the natives in West African had/have a lack of trust in international efforts to combat disease and Ebola.[16] Strangely, since the reported outbreaks of mass Ebola virus infections, some groups of native Africans have expressed doubt that Ebola really exists. Others have voiced allegations that health officials purposely infected the populations to harvest their organs. Hospitals, health care stations and workers have been attacked and stoned by mobs. Awareness, quarantine, and prohibition of touching people sick or dead from the disease have been viewed by many Africans as myths of Western propaganda. The African custom of touching and washing the body of a dead person prior to burial was being denied and led to resentment, demonstrations, and riots. Further, such public health measures are alien to their culture. Many West Africans believe in cultural superstitions and view Ebola as a curse rather than a pathogen, associating Ebola with witchcraft and sorcery brought there by foreigners. Some locals believe that doctors are killing Ebola patients as a punishment for sexual promiscuity. Fabio Friscia, UNICEF coordinator of the Ebola awareness campaign explained that what was creating the greatest problem in controlling Ebola was the "behavior of the population."

In Guinea, Liberia, and Sierra Leone the local population often attacked and disrupted health care workers, forcing them to leave treatment centers and hospitals. In one episode occurring in South-East Guinea, eight members of an Ebola disinfection and awareness team were killed with stones and machetes by fearful villagers. The members killed were part of a relief wing of the Christian and Missionary Alliance.

In August of 2014, armed locals attacked a medical clinic in Liberia, in an area named West Point, where patients were quarantined. Locals broke down doors, stole bloody mattresses, sheets, and equipment and caused patients to flee in a panic. The day before the raid, a crowd of several hundred locals drove away burial teams and police, chanting "No Ebola in West Point."

Violent attacks have resulted in Doctors Without Borders and medical volunteers having to withdraw from their posts because of concerns for their safety. A spokesperson for Doctors Without Borders stated, "We understand very well that people are afraid because it is a new disease here, but these are not favorable working conditions so we are suspending our activities."

Despite such difficult times, the story of ZMapp is not over. As both foreign as well as African health care providers and doctors continued to die from Ebola virus infection, the WHO endorsed the use of ZMapp to combat the uncontrollable outbreak. Liberian President, Ellen Johnson Sirleaf, in a direct request to President Obama, asked for a supply of the drug to be used for the treatment of local doctors.

Representing the producers of ZMapp, a spokesperson for Kentucky BioProcessing stated,"Though this is all relatively new and there's still a long way to go and a lot of things are going to happen as we go into drug-approval protocols with ZMapp…I think certainly it shows great promise that the tobacco plant can be utilized for such things. We'll see where that goes. We're certainly optimistic." Chapter 10 of this book will reveal if that optimism is justified.

Robert Garry: Managing the Effort to Curtail Ebola's Curse

O n 24th May 2014, the first person suspected of carrying Ebola arrived at KGH in Sierra Leone. The patient, a woman, had suffered a miscarriage and was clinically sick with bleeding and a high fever while complaining of a headache and backache. She had recently attended the funeral of a traditional healer, who was well-known in the area for her treatments and medicinal skills that cured local diseases.[1] The healer had been administering individuals from Guinea suffering from the symptoms of hemorrhagic fever. Soon afterward, she became ill herself and died.

Physicians at KGH knew of the Ebola outbreak raging in Guinea, although no-one they knew of had yet been affected in Sierra Leone. Nevertheless, precautions were taken at KGH in case individuals infected with Ebola were to cross the shared border of Guinea/Sierra Leone. The previous March, Kristian Andersen of Harvard/MIT's Broad Institute had set up testing with PCR (polymerase chain reaction), a method of identifying viral DNA or RNA in blood. Anderson anticipated that Ebola infections occurring in Guinea would eventually appear in Sierra Leone, and this test would be ready to detect Ebola RNA. The wait was not long. Within just a few days after the diagnostic test for Ebola was designed and implemented at KGH, the "mysterious deadly infectious disease" occurring in Guinea was definitively shown to be Ebola.[2] That result was posted on the internet 23 March 2014, and the test was available at KGH within a few days. Two months later the woman who had had a miscarriage, and first suspected infected patient, arrived at KGH. A sample of her blood was tested by Augustine Goba and was positive for the Ebola virus infection.[3] A portion of the blood sample sent to the Broad Institute was subsequently confirmed by Pardis Sabeti's group there as containing Ebola virus. The patient was promptly placed in the KGH Lassa isolation ward. Information about this first confirmed Ebola patient in Sierra Leone reached Bob Garry in the U.S. Garry was the person largely responsible for set-up, maintenance and training at the Lassa fever ward while working with Sheik Khan. Garry was also in charge of maintaining the diagnostic and research infrastructure at KGH and in the surrounding Sierra Leone area. He rapidly left New Orleans, arriving at KGH to ensure that the staff was prepared, properly outfitted with protective garments and using masks. He began collecting blood to be used for diagnosis of patients as well as preparation of samples to be sent to Sabeti's group for virus genome analysis. This procedure was accomplished at the start and throughout the Ebola rampage in the endangered African areas. The blood of infected victims contains high titers of Ebola virus, and contamination by this highly infectious agent can cause the specimen's handler to suffer a lethal outcome. After its collection from patients, such blood is treated with chemicals to inactivate the Ebola virus' infectivity but preserves sufficient viral RNA for sequencing and serum proteins for analysis. In addition, these blood samples are studied to characterize the infected individual's immune response to the infection as well as to perform the chemical assays necessary to treat the patient and track his/her infection for clinical care. Samples sent out of Sierra Leone for analysis had to, first, pass a critical human subjects' review and then receive permission to exit the country by the KGH hospital committee and the Sierra Leone government. Bringing samples into the United States for analysis also required a comprehensive review by the CDC, NIH, and the institute where the samples would be sent before performing their specific assay. In this case, official approvals had been awarded to the Tulane Medical Center (the location of Garry's team for antibody analysis) and to the Harvard and MIT Broad Institute (Sabeti's team for viral genome analysis). Later, The Scripps Research Institute in La Jolla, California (Oldstone, Sullivan, and de la Torre teams) also received such approval from their institute's human subjects research review committee as well as from the NIH to study innate and adoptive immune responses of individuals infected by Ebola. Obtaining permission to ship and study samples has been and is labor- and time-intensive and requires persistent but competent workers who can tell a truthful and accurate story with appropriate details.[4,5] In terms of overall organization, Bob Garry was the right person at the right time to accomplish these details working with both African, American, WHO officials and representatives.

Bob Garry was born in Terre Haute, Indiana, obtained a Bachelor of Science degree in Life Sciences from Indiana State University and a Ph.D. in Microbiology from the University of Texas at Austin. After postdoctoral training and a junior faculty appointment in the Department of Microbiology, Garry was recruited to Tulane University School of Medicine at New Orleans, Louisiana, where he rose to Professor of Microbiology and Immunology and Director of the Interdisciplinary Program in Molecular and Cellular Biology.[5]

A major component of Garry's responsibility was managing a consortium of scientists who were and are developing countermeasures against African hemorrhagic viruses, including diagnostics, immunotherapeutic and vaccines. One of Garry's defining accomplishments was the development of immunoassays with high sensitivity and specificity for Ebola virus.[6] The Ebola rapid diagnostic test devised by Garry and colleagues was initially the only immunoassay to receive emergency use authorizations from both the FDA and WHO. "It's a rapid test that is able to indicate if the Ebola virus is present in 15 minutes or less. It's something we have been working on for several years with Lassa fever, so it was much easier to put together a program where we can develop the test which works very well," explained Garry. However, bureaucratic difficulties arose thus taking longer than necessary for the test to be used. Garry added "this test can really make a difference in containment by placing people in the right holding facilities. The WHO is now running a trial and it is working just the way we had hoped." "It's a rapid test that is able to indicate if the patient is or isn't affected."

The Eastern Province of Sierra Leone has the world's highest annual incidence of Lassa fever[7] and the largest number of persons infected with Ebola during the 2013-2016 outbreak.[8] KGH was an important site for clinical and laboratory research on Lassa fever throughout the 1970s and 1980s. The violent civil conflict, sometimes referred to as the Blood Diamonds War, broke out in 1991 and did not end until 2003.[9] This clash forced suspension of Lassa fever research that was being done at the CDC center set up at the Nixon Memorial Hospital at Segbwema, which is roughly 62 miles from Kenema. This field station and laboratory had been established by Joseph McCormick.[10] Because that site was unsafe for medical personnel during the civil war, part of the CDC's effort was moved to the KGH center in Sierra Leone. Following the cessation of hostilities, a consortium of Lassa fever researchers led by Garry began rebuilding the scientific infrastructure at KGH. Now, in response to the Ebola outbreak and in anticipation of a future epidemic, work began and is NOW completed on a new viral hemorrhagic fever (VHF) ward of 42 beds, an increase over the original 14 beds and with improved isolation units and patient waste disposal systems. The finished complex will be named the Khan Center of Excellence at KGH. This name celebrates the late Dr. Sheik Khan who was the director of the KGH Lassa ward and died there after contracting Ebola from his patients[11] (as described in Chapter 4). Because of its historic contributions to VHF research and the prominent role it played in the West African Ebola outbreak, KGH has been established as a Center of Excellence for work on VHFs. Presently, Bob Garry is Director of the International Center of Infectious Diseases Research. Through support of NIH's Human Health and Heredity Program (H3Africa) as well as the Wellcome Trust and World Bank, the KGH center is expanding training opportunities for West African scientists in infectious diseases and genomics research. Garry was also a member of the leadership teams that founded the Viral Hemorrhagic Fever Consortium (VHFC),[12] and the African Center of Excellence for Genomics of Infectious Diseases (ACEGID),[13] which is part of the H3Africa Consortium.[14]

The West African Ebola outbreak provided the opportunity to test the facilities and tests developed by Garry, Andersen, Sabeti, and their colleagues. The Ebola outbreak began in December 2013, originating in a region of forested Guinea located only about a three-hour drive from KGH. The identity of this fever was established by genome sequencing.[2,3] Sick individuals began arriving at the KGH Lassa Fever/ Ebola clinic two months later and provided, for the first time, an opportunity for analysis in an advanced clinical and laboratory infrastructure designed for thorough study of viral hemorrhagic fevers. There, diagnosis of the first case of Ebola in Sierra Leone emerged. In addition, VHFC scientists led by Pardis Sabeti at the Broad Institute received samples for analysis of Ebola virus genetics/genomics as the virus spread into and through

Sierra Leone.[3] That study demonstrated a single introduction of Ebola virus into a human recipient with subsequent human-to-human spread,[3] and documented a rapid accumulation of mutations in the viral genome. VHFC and others extended these studies by analyzing Ebola virus genetic variability as it spread through the populations of West Africa.[15] VHFC also performed the largest and most in-depth clinical study and provided the best written description of Ebola virus disease to date.[16] The clinical study showed that, in addition to the expected findings of fever, lethargy, and headache, this West African variant of Ebola virus caused a gastrointestinal illness that focused attention on a newfound clinical aspect of the disease. Bleeding manifestations that predominated in prior Ebola outbreaks in central Africa[17] occurred but with a lower frequency than before (~1% of patients). Basic studies of the gastrointestinal malfunction revealed that the Ebola virus delta peptide functioned as a viroporin or an enterotoxin with a likely role in Ebola virus pathogenesis. Thus, for the 2013-2016 Ebola outbreak, Garry's work with the Sabeti team was essential in determining where and when the viral spread took off. Genomic analysis of the Ebola viruses isolated throughout the outbreak documented that the incidences of Ebola during 2014 in Sierra Leone originated from the Ebola virus isolated earlier in Guinea.[2,3,18] Spread to humans in Sierra Leone came from individuals who performed the ritual their culture fostered, attending their traditional healer's funeral, but the consequence was migration of and the infection they carried to Sierra Leone. From there the virus spread uncontrollably throughout Sierra Leone. This conclusion was derived from amino acid sequences of 99 viral genomes from 78 Ebola-infected individuals.[3] Garry commented…"This is the first study to document deep viral genomics during a human outbreak of a hemorrhagic fever like Ebola." "We get a close look at not only how the virus is evolving as it passes from one person to the next, but also how the virus changes as it replicates within a person."

When information from the first patient with Ebola in Sierra Leone at KGH was known, Garry returned to KGH bringing 28 cases of personal protective equipment including full suits and face masks. All health care providers who see or treat Ebola infected patients must wear these items. Because the virus is so highly contagious ..."we tell them to wear gloves and to protect their eyes and we've shown people how to do a traditional burial, only wearing gloves. And you can allow the body to be washed briefly. Workers have been attentive to the traditions, allowing the body to be wrapped without exposing people to the virus"... Garry stated.

Sheik Khan and Garry had worked together for nearly 10 years and, over that time, developed both a professional and personal relationship. Khan was more than a colleague to Garry; he was a close friend. When speaking of his personality and work, Garry described Khan as "a national hero" and "tremendous human being." However, as Ebola's curse exponentially increased its spread in tandem with exposure to an over-worked and exhausted Khan, Garry pressed himself harder to find possible remedies. Simultaneously, he strove to raise awareness throughout the international community and to Americans as well as raising money, soliciting contributions for supplies, funding equipment, and attracting participation from physicians and nurses. Endlessly, he repeated, "We're working on vaccines and medicines for Ebola and other hemorrhagic fevers, the solutions are coming!"

As the outbreak spiraled out of control, Garry repeatedly traveled back and forth between the United States and KGH. "It's been an eventful six weeks. I would be going back (to KGH) except there are things that are needed that I can't do over there like be in communication with people who are funding the work and trying to get more funding and things like that." But in the end, the epidemic infected over 11,000 individuals in Sierra Leone. The epidemic was reported as dying out in 2015. However, several new cases occurred in 2016 as Ebola simmered along. The WHO Director General reported an end of the epidemic on 30 March 2016, since no new cases were reported for 42 days after the most recent cluster on 14 January 2016. However, Ebola had not finished its work. Sporadically, new cases subsequently occurred. Sheik Khan and many of his original health care staff would not be up front to see and care for these newly Ebola-infected individuals. Sheik Khan and over 40% of his health care providers died from the first round of the battle against Ebola in KGH. Let's hope that the United States government and other governments and organizations have not abandoned the battle against Ebola, and that they will not again engage too little or too late. That concern arises justifiably as $500 million dollars formerly appropriated for Ebola by the USA to control and better understand Ebola virus were recently withdrawn and sent to respond, instead, to Zika infection, despite Ebola's continued rumble in West Africa. The depletion of funds likely played a major role in unpreparedness when the large 2018-2020 outbreak of Ebola occurred in Central Africa (see chapter 10).

Garry had a deep personal and professional relationship with Khan. Their work together had substantial effects on how the Ebola outbreak played out. Garry managed the set-up and maintenance training at the Lassa virus ward with Khan and traveled back and forth to Sierra Leone and the US bringing necessary medication, gear and equipment. His work in countermeasures to control Ebola virus infection, including diagnostics, immune analysis and sample collection. Samples he and his colleagues collected were used for analysis of the virus' genetic structure and of the infected persons' innate and adoptive immune responses. This resulted in the success of a diagnostic test that swiftly detected Ebola virus in the blood of patients. Analysis of the Ebola virus's genome during the outbreak was then possible and supplied much needed information about the virus' spread and mutation frequency, the kinetics, strength of the immune response raised against the virus, and identities of viral sites recognized by antibodies and CTLs. Before, throughout, and after the Ebola outbreak, Garry was accompanied by Pardis Sabeti, who became a close friend and colleague.

Pardis Sabeti: Geneticist Tracking Ebola's Travels and Changing Profile

An operational Viral Hemorrhagic Fever Consortium group containing scientists and medical workers from Kenema Government Hospital (KGH), Tulane, Harvard/MIT plus others from West Africa and the United States was set up to combat and study Lassa fever virus [LASV] infection. The group included Sheik Khan, Robert Garry, and Pardis Sabeti in leadership roles.[1]

Pardis Sabeti, after her undergraduate training at the Massachusetts Institute of Technology, attended the University of Oxford where she obtained (in 2002) a Doctor of Philosophy degree in Biological Anthropology. Her work was on "The effects of natural selection and recombination on genetic diversity in humans." Her thesis investigated malaria in African populations. Her studies examined genetic diversity in Africans and host susceptibility to malaria.[1] Pardis developed new algorithms to study natural selection.[1] These studies helped prepare her for future investigations on Ebola in West Africa, which occurred after she attended and received a medical degree from Harvard in 2006. After graduating from medical school, Pardis took postdoctoral work that continued her prior studies under the mentorship of the well-known geneticist and molecular biologist Eric Lander, head of the MIT Broad Institute in Cambridge, Massachusetts. During her postdoctoral time, Pardis continued research focused on development of methodologies and software to detect natural selection in genome-wide studies and in scanning the human genome for evidence of natural selection in specific infectious diseases. Her academic accomplishments led to her recruitment for a faculty appointment at the Center for Systems Biology, Department of Organismic and Evolutionary Biology at the Broad Institute of MIT and Harvard in 2008. There, Pardis set up her own laboratory and worked to develop new analytic methods and use rapidly emerging genomic knowledge and resources to study evolutionary adaptation in humans and pathogens.[2,3] The idea was to investigate and characterize functional changes that shaped the responses of human species over time to selected human pathogens. Part of these studies led her to investigate the genetic diversity of LASV and how mutations in the infected host's cell receptor may account for human susceptibility or resistance to this virus. The receptor on the surface of the cell, in this case alpha-dystroglycan (a-DG), modified by the glycosyltransferase (enzyme) LARGE, leads to the LASV attachment to and entrance into the cell, where it can then replicate its progeny.[4,5] It was from her observations of mutations in LARGE occurring in epidemic areas of LASV infection that Pardis became more involved in countries in West Africa (Sierra Leone and Nigeria) where Lassa is endemic, and where she worked with the Viral Hemorrhagic Fever Consortium.[1] Pardis started work on LASV in 2008 at KGH both to help in the rapid diagnosis of individual patients as well as to uncover other pathogens.[1] The idea was to provide warnings of local outbreaks before these might become a global threat. Thus, the team of Sheik Khan, Bob Garry, and Pardis Sabeti was formed, joined with other colleagues, and traveled to Nigeria to inaugurate the African Center of Excellence for Genomics of Infectious Diseases. The Viral Hemorrhagic Fever Consortium was instrumental in setting up this Center in Ogun State, Nigeria, an epidemic area for LASV and LASV infection. The Center's mission was to monitor dangerous infectious agents in West Africa.[6]

It was the unexpected outbreak of Ebola starting in 2013 and peaking in 2014-2016 in Sierra Leone and other parts of West Africa that turned Dr Sabeti's attention and commitment to investigating the diversity in Ebola virus and examining how Ebola evolved in terms of an infectious agent causing such profound morbidity, mortality, and misery in humans. To quote the father of microbiology, Louis Pasteur ..."Chance favors the prepared mind."

A vivacious, intelligent, and determined scientific explorer, Pardis' American adventure began when she and her family fled the Iranian revolution in 1979, emigrating from Iran at age 2. In a whirlwind of academic achievements followed, during her early years of academic life. Prior to her 40TH birthday, she was awarded a Rhodes Scholarship (1997-2000), Burroughs Wellcome Fund Career Award in the Biomedical Sciences (2006-2013), and a recent Howard Hughes Medical Institute Investigator Award (2015-on). She received the Ellis Island Medal of Honor (2013), Carnegie Corporation of New York Great Immigrants Award (2014), the Smithsonian magazine's American Ingenuity Award in the Natural Sciences (2012), National Geographic Emerging Explorer Award (2013), and for her work on Ebola she was named one of TIME Magazine's Persons of the Year in 2014 (Ebola Fighters) and one of TIME Magazine's 100 most influential people in 2015.[7] In addition to her life in science and teaching, Pardis is an active musician. Remarkably, she was and continues as the lead singer and bass player of the rock band "Thousand Days" that she helped form.

The band received an Honorable Mention in the Billboard World Song Contest. The band and Pardis, besides performing and composing albums, also made/make music videos to spark and enlighten young people's interest and knowledge in science.[8]

Her work to determine whether a specific genetic variation in a given host gene is widespread in a population as a result of favored natural selection against a pathogen involves analysis and understanding factors that influence the response of humans to the pathogen under scrutiny as well as the genome of the pathogen. This is challenging work and in part is reflective of the influence of her father, Parviz Sabeti, who was a high-ranking official in the late Shah of Iran's government and known for taking tough, meaningful jobs. According to Pardis ..."(he) took one of the toughest jobs in the Iranian government because he cared about his nation more than himself... his courage and conviction have always driven me to want to make a difference -- making the world a better place".[7] Thus, Pardis led a team to sequence the viral genome (Ebola and Lassa) from infected individuals at the beginning and during the infectious outbreaks. She was one of the first to use in-depth real-time DNA sequencing in the midst of a deadly epidemic.[9]

Obtaining 99 samples from 78 different patients in the first three weeks of the Ebola outbreak in Sierra Leone at KGH,[9] Sabeti and her colleagues showed genetic similarity between viruses sequenced at Sierra Leone compared to sequences from Ebola viruses isolated at Guinea where in 2013 the outbreak began. The results suggested the epidemic started with a single transmission into the human population from a natural animal reservoir and then continued by human-to-human transmission (see Figure 2).[9,10] The human-to-human transmission both continued and extended the outbreak. These results reinforced the medical and public health need to reduce human-to-human contact while providing the rationale to do so.

Later sequencing data obtained on analysis of Ebola genome

from 232 blood samples taken over a seven-month period in Sierra Leone led Sabeti and colleagues to confirm that one form of virus entered the country and continued to spread. Further, the earlier genetic versions of Ebola genome in Guinea did not go away, that is were not replaced by selective mutations, but instead continued to spread within Guinea to its capital city, Conakry, population over 1,668,000 people. Ebola virus isolated and sequenced in Conakry continued to be the close version of Ebola first isolated in Guinea and Sierra Leone.[9,10] Thus, the early lineage "A Ebola virus" was persisting again pointing to the fact that all virus samples apparently descended from one source. All told, the accumulated data strongly indicated that the entire outbreak was likely caused by an introduction of a single virus from an animal reservoir. Despite border closings among neighboring West African countries monitored by local police, soldiers, and WHO, sick people from the Taï Forest area continued to cross back and forth into and out of Guinea to Sierra Leone and to Liberia.[11] The Taï Forest borders the west coasts of Guinea, Sierra Leone, and Liberia. When a second wave of infected individuals emerged as, border crossing and migration of people continued unchecked, the number of individuals infected exceeded that comprising the first wave. Health officials in Guinea and at WHO knew sick people had crossed into Sierra Leone in March 2014 since discovery of the first case in Guinea in December 2013. Illness from Ebola was not detected in Sierra Leone until May 2014. The first laboratory diagnosis of Ebola in Sierra Leone was made in May 2014 at KGH when a blood sample from an ill individual was tested for viral RNA. For this test, parts of the RNA from the Ebola virus was used with RNA isolated from the patient's blood to see if the sample contained RNA identical to that of the Ebola virus. This assay is called a polymerase chain reaction (PCR). The PCR test was set-up in March in anticipation that Ebola raging in Guinea might/would soon occur in Sierra Leone. This came to pass, and the positive diagnosis led Sabeti to set up and send a team with advanced diagnostic skills and equipment to KGH. The object was to assist in rapid analysis of the genomic sequence of Ebola to study its spread and evolution. Pardis commented, "The faster you can get a diagnosis of Ebola, the faster you can stop it...the big question is, is this going to be stopped?"

Attending a single funeral where numerous people were exposed to Ebola was the start of the Ebola epidemic in Sierra Leone. By touching and washing the body of the dead local shaman, numerous individuals became infected. "Virus like a tidal wave was coming into the country (Sierra Leone)..."the first case was manageable" lamented Pardis. Virus infections were expanding exponentially with a doubling period of 35 days. Concern was to prevent Ebola from migrating to larger cities where large susceptible populations lived: Conakry in Guinea (over 1,667,000 population), Freetown in Sierra Leone (nearly 1,000,000), Monrovia in Liberia (over 1,000,000) and Lagos in Nigeria (over 17,000,000). Questions arose early from those involved in fighting to combat and stop the spread of the infection. First, were new Ebola virus variants developing that would increase the human host range and have the ability to cause more severe or less severe human disease? Second, was the human immune response to fight the virus being compromised? The immune response could be compromised by several different mechanisms. For example, Ebola might suppress the ability of the host's immune response to recognize and combat the virus. Ebola might by mutation change its own amino acids to avoid recognition by the host's immune response, i.e., Ebola variants that escape either virus-specific T cell recognition or virus-specific antibody recognition, the pillars of the adoptive immune response. The virus might influence the production of interferon (type 1), an early innate host response made by the infected person to limit (interfere) with virus spread and protect uninfected cells from being invaded by the virus. Interferon is known to be suppressed by one of Ebola virus' proteins, VP35. Alternatively, might Ebola virus cause an exaggerated excessive immune response that could enhance anti-Ebola T cell numbers and responses leading to an event known as "cytokine storm." The end result of cytokine storm is attracting the body's scavenger and killer cells which results in their causing increased injury of tissues and killing of both Ebola infected cells and non-infected host cells. This is called immunopathology. As is known for other viral infections, virus-induced immunopathology can enhance the clinical symptoms (what the patient feels and states) and signs (what the doctor finds and describes) by injuring tissues and cells as a consequence of an exaggerated antiviral immune response. Cytokine storm is the excessive release of small protein molecules called cytokines or chemokines known to, through a variety of chemical reactions to attract macrophages, polymorphonuclear cells, and lymphocytes to a site. Interaction of these programmed host cells with infected and non-infected cells can cause enhanced morbidity and mortality from the virus infection. Cytokine storm has also been suspected of playing a role during acute Ebola infection as shown in animal models and by high levels of cytokines/chemokines in infected humans. In addition, anti-Ebola viral antibodies alone or with participation of cells that bear Fc receptors or with the participation of complement proteins can also cause tissue and cell injury.

With all eyes on the West African outbreak raging in 2014, Ebola infection erupted concurrently in Central Africa. In July 2014, Ebola reappeared in Central Africa, where it had been first recorded in 1976. This outbreak occurred in the Democratic Republic of the Congo (DRC) in 2014 in the rural village of Inkanamongo, which is located in the vicinity of Boende. Of the 66 cases there were 49 deaths for a mortality rate of 74%. Among the dead were eight health care workers. Inkanamongo is located in a humid, tropical forest delineated by two large rivers and with poor roads in and out. At the time, this was the seventh Ebola outbreak in DRC. By 2020, DRC recorded 12 outbreaks of Ebola. By contrast, over 28,000 cases of Ebola-Zaire, the largest burst yet recorded occurred in West Africa in 2013-2016. Interestingly, the Ebola-Zaire virus isolated from this 2014 outbreak in DRC was 99% identical to other Ebola-Zaire viruses isolated in the DRC years earlier, and more than 97% identical to Ebola viruses isolated in 2014 and 2015 from Sierra Leone.[9,12] How an almost identical Ebola-Zaire viral strain from the Congo in Central Africa could also be found in West Africa is unclear as the area is separated by over 2,400 miles. Independent earlier studies by D.W. Thomas of the University of Aberdeen and Heidi Richter of the University of Florida used tagging collars and satellite tracking of fruit bats in Central Africa. Their results showed that bats could cover 621 miles of territory during a one-month period. One bat named "Hercules" was recorded to have flown 1,180 miles journey in six months. The majority of tagged bats were never found, likely owing to a high mortality during their travels. There are two favored general theories in an attempt to explain how a similar Ebola virus strain could appear in two such distant areas.[13,14] It is highly unlikely that a single bat could travel the 2,400-mile distance from the Congo to Guinea/Sierra Leone. The first hypothesis is that migration of fruit bats to one area infects other fruit bats in a more distant area. Like a relay race, an infected bat in the Congo infects a bat along the way and this bat continues to pass on the virus to other susceptible bats until one reaches West Africa. A second hypothesis is that some endogenous fruit bats in and residing around the Taï Forest carrying the Ebola-Taï Forest strain while other fruit bats in the forest are carriers of the Ebola-Zaire virus. The Taï Forest borders on the west coast of Guinea, Liberia, and Sierra Leone, and the Ivory Coast countries and harbors fruit bats, many bird species, pygmy hippopotamus, leopards, and monkeys, including chimpanzees. It was from a dead chimpanzee found in the Taï Forest that at autopsy infected the one and only prior case of Ebola in West Africa prior to the 2013-2016 outbreak. The Ebola virus recovered from the Ebola-Taï Forest virus has about a 65%

sequence homology with Ebola-Zaire viruses isolated from the Congo or isolated from Sierra Leone or Guinea. Hence, they are very different Ebola virus strain. Perhaps both species of Ebola viruses exist in different bat populations living in the Taï Forest. The continued encroachment by natives into the Tai forest may have led then to exposure of one or more individuals to the Zaire-Ebola strain. Although many suspect the bats as a primary source of Ebola, full-length infectious virus, at this time, no such sample has been isolated from these mammals. Rather, Ebola RNA or antibodies to Ebola are their current signatures. So, for Pardis Sabeti, the scientific investigators, and the world community the mystery of what primary host carries this virus that infects humans still awaits solving.

Ebola's Curse: Impact
on the Economics
of West Africa

D uring the Great Depression, Franklin Delano Roosevelt, the 32nd US president used his inaugural address in 1932 to rally Americans by saying "The only thing we have to fear, is fear itself." Indeed, fear of death, of being infected or of not finding a safe haven to save one's life played a major role in the West African Ebola epidemic of 2013-2016. This was reflected by Ebola's pivotal role in unraveling the economy of West Africa. As stated by the World Bank, "The largest economic effects of the crisis are not the direct costs (mortality, morbidity, caregiving, and the associated losses of working days- but rather those resulting from changes in behavior-driven by fear which have resulted in generally lower demands for goods and services and consequently lower domestic income and employment".[1]

An example of the environment of fear was recorded by J. Daniel Kelly in a personal note he published in the journal *Nature* on his experience of first going to Africa and witnessing

Ebola.[1] "I will never forget the first time I walked into an Ebola isolation ward at Connaught Hospital in Freetown, Sierra Leone. It was 20 August 2014. Inside, eight people thought to have the disease were organized into three patient-care rooms. Patients in the first room appeared to be healthy, and we greeted each other. In the second room, patients barely had the strength to sit. Still, they were able to articulate how they felt. In the last room there were two patients. One was a woman who seemed confused and agitated and was later confirmed to have the disease. On the other side of the room, a young man was curled into the corner of his bed. He seemed healthy but was terrified. He had been deathly ill when he was admitted three days earlier. He recovered but had watched Ebola kill two others in that room."

"I could only imagine how I would feel in that situation, watching others get sick and die, wondering if I would be next. Then I considered the deplorable conditions -- no visitors were allowed, and a bucket served as a bathroom -- and how I, wearing my protective 'spacesuit', must have looked to the curled man. The idea of becoming sick with Ebola in Sierra Leone frightened me."

"It frightened him too, and much of his fear could have been avoided. It took four days for his blood to be tested and shown to be free of Ebola. At that point, Sierra Leone had two facilities able to diagnose the virus. The nearest -- Kenema Government Hospital -- was five hours away and was overloaded with blood samples from around the country."

"The Sierra Leonean doctor who had (recently) supervised the ward had died, and no Sierra Leonean doctor had taken his place. The man was locked in this terrifying environment until someone could draw his blood for testing. Blood samples and sick patients were sent to Kenema by ambulance only at the end of each day. Even after the man's blood sample arrived in Kenema, it was not tested until the next day...".

"People who think that they might have the disease do not want to spend several days trapped in an isolation unit, away from their families and surrounded by workers in spacesuits. This fear means that patients go to isolation wards only when their symptoms are severe, if they go at all."

The 2013-2016 Ebola outbreak in Sierra Leone had and continues to have a drastic negative effect on its economy as well as the economies of Guinea and Liberia. Before Ebola, all these West African countries recorded substantial growth and had overcome most of the economic strain of the recent civil war. In 2013 Sierra Leone and Liberia were ranked second and sixth among the top 10 countries with the highest GDP growth in the world. GDP subsequently fell as Ebola expanded. World Bank President Jim Yong Kim stated, "Ebola's potential inflicted massive economic costs on Guinea, Liberia, and Sierra Leone and on the rest of their neighbors in west Africa."[1]

Ebola cost Sierra Leone the largest decrease in its GDP. Before the Ebola outbreak in 2014, growth was at 11.3% but by end of 2014 it decreased to 8%. Ebola infections spread to 12 of the 13 districts in Sierra Leone leaving a substantial trail of economic disruption and deaths.[1] Most involved were the eastern provinces where Sierra Leone borders Guinea and Liberia. Sierra Leone's Minister of Agriculture, Joseph Sam Sesay, told the BBC on 9 October 2015, that cabinet discussions with President Ernest Bai Koroma revealed a fall in the country's total economy of the country fell by over 30%.[2] Agriculture, the most important economic category endured the greatest impact, since, about 66% of the working population were farmers. Road- blocks were set-up by police and military as recommended by the Chief Coordinator for the United Nations Development Program (UNDP) and public health officials to prevent migration of infected individuals from spreading the Ebola infection to uninfected persons. However, the road blocks also prevented the movement of farmers, other laborers, supplies, shipments of goods and farm produce.[5]

Farms were abandoned by people scared of contracting Ebola, as they ran away to less diseased areas. Consequently, no planting was done for the next year's future crops. About 80 percent of farmers reported that their harvest was smaller than the previous year.[2,7] Unfortunately hardly any food had been stored as insurance against future famine. The result was higher food prices and a rise in inflation. Many families could not afford the costly staples. As an example, roughly two-thirds of households were not able to purchase enough rice for their needs.[1] The avalanche of difficulties and troubles steam-rolled onward, leading to a shortage of money for foreign exchange, a disrupted and angered population, slowdown in transportation services, and a halt in building operations. Further, the service sector suffered from a migration out of the area by foreign workers whose spending in Sierra Leone, Guinea, and Liberia was an important part of the economy.[1,6,7] These cataclysmic economic events caused commercial banks to reduce the granting of loans and capital funding. Bank hours were reduced, usually by half or more, both for economic reasons and fear of contact with those infected with Ebola. The tourist industry suffered greatly. Hotels were empty or closed. Staff was laid off. Multiple airlines suspended flights in and out of Sierra Leone and Liberia as the tourist trade dropped and for fear of viral infection. Limiting air flights compromised the delivery into Ebola virus infected areas of medical supplies and volunteer health care workers.[7,8] In all, closure of borders and suspension of air flights limited the abilities of Ebola-infected countries to export and import, thereby severely hampering their economies.

Ebola directly compromised the booming mining industry in Sierra Leone, Liberia, and Guinea.[9] Mining had accounted for a large part of the country's recent growth potential. Especially hard hit were the world's largest steel maker, ArcelorMittal in Liberia, and iron ore mining operations in Guinea. Closure of mining companies, impairment of services, and depletions in the agriculture sector led to a decline in Guinea's predicted growth rate of 4.5% at the beginning of 2014, falling to 2.4% in the next six months.[10,11]

West African countries rely heavily on agriculture for their GDP and suffered greatly when that sector became impaired. According to the local Food and Agriculture Organization, agriculture accounts for 57% of Sierra Leones GDP, 39% of Liberia's, and 20% of Guinea's.[1] Many farmers fled their farms for fear that the virus would reach them. Sierra Leone's Agriculture Minister Joseph Sam Sesay stated, "We are definitely expecting a devastating effect not only on labor availability and capacity but we are also talking about farms being abandoned by people running away from the epicenters and going to areas that don't have the disease."[5] With the abandonment of a large numbers of farms, the food supply decreased and food prices increased. David Evans, a senior economist of The World Bank stated, "Three-quarters of the households in Liberia are reporting significant food insecurity;" Liberia's price per rice bag increased from $28 to $35. Guinea has seen the largest loss in its agriculture industry since it is one of the world's top producers of coca and palm oil.[11]

Ebola struck during the planting season, disrupting the planting and growing of stable crops such as rice and maize, leading to significant food shortages. Chief co-coordinator for the United Nations Development Programme, David McLachlann-Karr elaborated, "We are now coming into the planting season which means a lot of agriculture is not happening, so down the line that will create food shortages and pressures on food prices. We are starting to see a rise in inflation and pressure on the national currency as well as a shortage of foreign exchange."[5] Farmers who comprised a majority of the population suffered greatly. Rural families had always depended on theses crops for both food and income.

Ebola made Sierra Leone, Guinea, and Liberia poorer in other ways. International investors downgraded these countries' potential for growth and investments dropped sharply as due the Ebola outbreak ragged. The World Bank reported on 7 October 2014, less than halfway into the Ebola epidemic, that the economic loss caused by Ebola virus infections across Sierra Leone, Guinea, and Liberia would likely reach US\$ 32.6 billion by the end of 2015.[10-12]

The severity of the Ebola epidemic led many non-African countries to become concerned about their exposure to the virus and the virus' transit into their homelands. Heightened control of visitors from West Africa and enhanced national security followed. The international community recognized that the outbreak was a global threat, not just a regional one. To contain the outbreak to Africa and prevent Ebola's spread elsewhere, international funding supported efforts to control the infection in Sierra Leone, Guinea, and Liberia. The UN stated that US\$1 billion was needed to restrict further outbreaks, whereas the World Bank estimated it could be billions.[11,12] Pledges arrived from several countries as well as from multilateral, bilateral, and private organizations. International donors including the World Bank and International Monetary Fund gave approximately US\$530 million to the countries hit the hardest. The US provided \$174 million in funding and sent 3,000 military troops to build treatment units for assistance in containing the outbreak. Money was also used for humanitarian support, medical supplies, and screening facilities at borders, airports and seaports, as well as strengthening the surveillance and treatment capacity of health systems. The African Union, adjacent African countries, and the African business community funded efforts to limit Ebola's spread to Nigeria, Cote d'Ivoire, Guinea-Bissau, Senegal and the Gambia. However, in 2015 a new outbreak of Ebola occurred in Central Africa, resulting in a reduction of aid provided by the African Union. Other European and Asian countries as well as Canada pledged funds, Cuba offered more than 460 doctors and health care workers.[13]

When summarizing why the Ebola outbreak caused such great economic damage, Finance Minister Amara Konneh of Liberia reported that the fall in GDP was caused by "damage done to mining, agriculture and service industries, loss of foreign workers, borders closing, and suspension of international flights."[14] Ebola virus further weakened the economy as infections spread and the government restricted mobility, trade, and transportation. Additionally, direct costs for health care to fight Ebola were substantial and funds insufficient. Other destabilizing events were lower labor productivity and unemployment. The accumulative result was an increased cost of doing business within these Ebola-infected countries, coupled with the fear of becoming infected, which led the populace to flee farms, factories, banks, and mining companies.

Once the Ebola outbreak was recognized, the Sierra Leone government placed restrictions on people crossing the borders. Cote d'Ivoire and Senegal followed by imposing restrictions on the movement of people and goods by closing their borders. Countries throughout Africa banned citizens of the three countries most ravaged by Ebola (Guinea, Sierra Leone, and Liberia) from entering their countries and prohibited their citizens from traveling to high risk areas of Ebola infection. These travel restrictions resulted in many migrant workers losing jobs and businesses along borders closing. Quarantine areas were created where outsiders were not allowed to enter. Regulators of the United Nations Development Programme (UNDP) believed roadblocks were required to containing the outbreak. The downside was that roadblocks also caused food shortages leading to further public dissatisfaction and protest. Chief co-coordinator of the UNDP stated that "A robust response to quarantining epicenters of the disease is absolutely necessary" but admitted that it has had devastating effects on the agriculture sector.[15]

Sierra Leone, Guinea, and Liberia also suffered from trade restrictions imposed from other African countries. Cross border trade accounted for from 20-75% of the GDP for West African countries.[16] Countries that traded with Sierra Leone, Guinea, and Liberia soon reduced or completely stopped such trade. Nearby countries in West Africa where Ebola had not surfaced such as the Ivory Coast and Senegal also lost trade, exports, and imports stemming from the fear that their exported products might be infected.

Similarly, small local community businesses were negatively impacted because of the restrictions, fear of disease, and decrease in consumers. To survive economically, businesses that were able to stay open reduced staff and working hours. The reduction of available funds also cut local spending of public funds that had been used for investment in physical capital [machines, equipment] and human capital [labor force]. These expenditures were reduced, deleted or decreased. Moreover, the decreased supply of available labor compromised businesses. The World Bank stated that during the outbreak "half of male heads of households (46%) in Liberia who were working prior to the epidemic remain unemployed, and even more (60%) of female household heads are out of work… and the country's primary productivity has been cut in half."[17]

The direct impact on tourism from Ebola's presence was manifested markedly when British Airways, Emirates, Air France, Asky Airlines and Arik Air implemented bans on most flights to and from the affected countries. According to Brookings, "CEOs eleven firms operating in West Africa have said that some measures, including these travel restrictions, are doing more harm than good and may well be contributing to the humanitarian crisis by blocking crucial trade flows, thereby pushing up the prices of essential foods and medicines". Some examples are the temporary closure of Cameroon's border with Nigeria and the announcement by Kenya Airways that it was suspending all flights to and from Sierra Leone and Liberia.[8,18]

Ebola's presence severely downgraded foreign investments. As international investors grew cautious, they scaled down foreign outlays leading to a decline of revenue and stability. According to broadcasts from Voice of America, investor confidence had dropped since the escalation of Ebola's impact. Foreign mining corporations such as China Union dramatically scaled down their operations in Liberia.[9] The majority of foreign investments in Sierra Leone, Liberia, and Guinea were in these countries' natural resources, many of which are limited or rare to find on other continents. However, when Ebola appeared many multi-national corporations decided making foreign investments was unprofitable. The increased death rate and quarantine closures increased unemployment, and the lack of available workers made it difficult for corporations to continue running their daily operations. Some miners were afraid to return to work in high-risk districts and simply quit their jobs. Others fled the area. Sierra Leone relies on mining for 17% of its GDP, and Liberia 14% of its GDP.[1] Firms including the Australian mining firm Tawana Resources and Canadian Overseas Petroleum Limited suspended their operations, sent foreign workers home. This pattern was repeated with other mining companies such as Simandou, Rio Tinto (the world's largest mining company), and London Mining.

The decline in economic activity led to a decline in fiscal revenues as revenues from taxes, tariffs and customs vanished. The World Bank found that short-term fiscal impacts were large, at $93 million for Liberia (4.7% of GDP); $79 million for Sierra Leone (1.8% of GDP); and $120 million for Guinea (1.8% of GDP).

In summary, the Ebola outbreak devastated the economies of Sierra Leone, Guinea, and Liberia.[1,4] Ebola led to restrictions on movements of people and goods, lack of investment and increasing costs of the health care. Mobility restrictions included closing the borders, shutting down businesses, diminished banking, and disrupted tourism. Such events led to accelerated and enhanced unemployment. Foreign trade and investments were aborted or slowed down. All these factors created stress on government revenues leading to inflation. The Ebola infected countries rely heavily on agriculture and mining, and their partial or complete shutdowns had devastating effects on jobs, employment, and government resources. Mining companies ended their operations and sent workers home. Farmers fled during planting season causing a future food shortage and increasing inflation. Fear of the virus, lack of education, and loss of communication played major roles in depression of the economy.[1,9] The WHO and international community once alerted attempted to help, but their commitment was overall insufficient and tardy. Thus, poor public health knowledge, delay in government and international response, and limited cooperation were all complicit in allowing a preventable disease to accelerate its spread from a few hundred to 28,000 cases and leading to economic disaster for the Ebola infected countries.

The Ebola outbreak was costly in many ways. Understanding what happened. and what needs to be done now show how to prevent another uncontrolled outbreak with resultant human suffering. The international response must be quicker and more serious. The first Ebola case occurred in Guinea in December 2013, in Sierra Leone in March 2014, and Doctors Without Borders were not notified or operational until two months later, in May 2014. The WHO waited until five months after the Ebola virus infection began and spread to declare a worldwide disaster, a delay likely due to the wrong person as the WHO's head at the wrong time. In contrast to the Ebola outbreak of 2013-2016, the WHO has the right person in charge and was effective in its response for handling the first pandemic of the 21st century, SARS.[20] Ebola also teaches that healthcare workers were under-equipped and limited, and that the basic healthcare structure needs to be built-up, strengthened and maintained. Education and protective clothing are imperative. Over 800 healthcare workers were infected and over 500 died. Also imperative is rapid surveillance followed by quarantine when appropriate. Finally, the political structure needs to understand and pay attention to the history of viral infection and communicate those facts, so all individuals and community leaders can trust their local and national governments.

Ebola's Arrival in West Africa (2013-2016) and its Scorecard: Failure of the World Health Organization and the International Community. Design of a World Health Plan to Abort Future Catastrophe

The international health community and its institutions made a slate of errors, each of which prolonged, helped to spread, and continued the Ebola epidemic from 2013 onward until its termination in 2016. Their failure took the form of responding too slowly, too inefficiently, and too ineffectively. When they did respond, international organizations such as the World Health Organization, World Bank and United Nations failed in their communications among one another, a major cause for delay of effective action needed to contain the viral disease. Non-governmental organizations clashed with the WHO and World Bank; the result was confusion about what was going on, what to do, or who was to do what. Multinational corporations (NGOs) initially contributed little of substance. Here, we describe the faults that caused such damage for the purpose of recommending steps to correct the errors and ensure that a catastrophe like this is less likely to occur in the future.

The WHO has its share of blame and rightly so. Its chartered role is to protect the health of our world's human populations, and its task is to live up to that purpose. It's major failure in the Ebola epidemic was in not understanding the public health disaster as it was unfolding, not placing enough people in the areas of involvement, and thus not acting early enough to limit the spread of Ebola virus infection. During the initial months of Ebola's debut, the WHO was slow in acknowledging that a unique infectious disease was advancing and killing people. Throughout this indolent period, Ebola continued to spread from Guinea across neighboring countries, primarily Sierra Leone and Liberia. With optimal public health control, the numbers of infections and deaths might have been 10-fold fewer or less, i.e., 28,000 to 2,800 and 11,300 to 1,300. Compared to the WHO's successes in handling prior epidemics of H1N1 and H5N1 influenza and SARS, the Ebola epidemic was largely ignored and handled poorly. The major cause of this failure by the WHO was mainly its administration at the time. Neither their personnel nor that of the international disease control community was sufficiently decisive in understanding, acting, or supervising the outbreak. "We can mount a highly effective response to small and medium-size outbreaks, but when faced with an emergency of this scale, our current systems -- national and international -- simply have not coped," stated WHO Director-General Margaret Chan, Deputy Director-General Anarfi Asamoa-Baah, and the organization's regional directors in a joint statement on April 16, 2016.[1] During the early phase of Ebola's outbreak, those in charge at WHO rarely left Geneva to travel to Guinea to actually see the unfolding catastrophe reported by Doctors without Borders or organizing the assistance requested. Of course, the earlier an infection is contained, the less likely it will spread from a small to a large problem. The WHO admitted it was ill prepared. "We have taken serious note of the criticisms that the initial WHO response was slow and insufficient, we were not aggressive in alerting the world ... we did not work effectively in coordination with other partners, there were shortcomings in risk communications and there was confusion of roles and responsibilities."[1] In contrast, the WHO led by a different administration in 2002-2004 acted forcefully and correctly when faced with the outbreak and possible pandemic effect of SARS (Severe Acute Respiratory Syndrome).[1]

The WHO was also defective in monitoring the Ebola outbreak. A critique by a group of twenty experts from the Harvard Global Health Institute and the London School of Hygiene and Tropical Medicine found that "The lack of capacity in Guinea to detect the virus for several months was a key failure, allowing Ebola eventually to spread to bordering Liberia and Sierra Leone, underscoring inadequate communication and arrangements between governments and the WHO to share, validate, and respond robustly to information on outbreak."[4] Indeed, after Ebola was initially identified, it still spread through the capital cities of Guinea and Liberia, and within two months appeared in other major cities and their international airports. Without protocols for identification of Ebola in place, the virus rapidly spread. The *RT International* report of November 23, 2015 stated, "Without any approved drugs, vaccines or rapid diagnostic tests, health workers struggled to diagnose patients and provide effective care. Without sufficient protective gear, and initially without widespread understanding of the virus, hundreds of health workers themselves became ill and died."[1]

In summary, early in the course of the Ebola infection, before its massive outbreak, Doctors Without Borders warned the

WHO about the potential threat. This evaluation, despite its highly qualified source, was originally disputed by the WHO. As a result, actions to fight the infection and arrange for humanitarian aid were delayed. Not until August 2014, a good eight months after the initial Ebola cases emerged in Guinea, did the WHO begin to act. The Harvard Global Health Institute's report called for greater accountability and transparency within all global health institutions and remarked that the WHO should respond to freedom of information requests.

In the West African countries, consistently poor health care and lack of adequate infrastructure were major factors in the increasing difficulty of addressing public health concerns and medical emergencies. By comparison, in Boston, at Peter Bent Brigham Hospital part of Harvard's medical complex, more physicians worked on the second floor alone than in all of Liberia. Most of the health care staff in countries overrun with Ebola virus infections was not sufficiently trained to respond. They often lacked even the basic materials required for treatment and had insufficient knowledge or equipment to protect themselves from contamination. The exceptions in some areas included Kenema Government Hospital in Sierra Leone and centers where Doctors Without Borders were located. For example, Dr. Mariano Lugli, a deputy director of operations for Doctors Without Borders, did respond to an early incidence of Ebola virus infection. Working in remote forests of Guinea during March 2014, when the outbreak spread to Guinea's capital, Conakry, Lugli set up a healthcare receiving and treatment clinic. Although Lugli was met by a foreign medic and logistician sent by the UN health agency, he never saw or met a WHO official who was responsible for handling this escalation of the outbreak. Lugli elaborates, "In all the meetings I attended, even in Conakry, I never saw a representative of the WHO. The coordination role the WHO should be playing, we just didn't see it. I didn't see it the first three weeks and we didn't see it afterwards."[1]

Because so many patients and their healthcare providers had already died and those not yet infected feared the same fate, many hospitals were shut down and abandoned. Hundreds of patients remained waiting in front of non-functional hospitals in the hope of being admitted and treated. The WHO received extensive criticism for taking too long to provide and organize the flow of physicians, healthcare workers, protective clothing, and even fluids. Without leadership by the WHO in pursuing outside governments and philanthropies to establish isolation centers, surveillance, and laboratory capacity in West Africa, the local governments turned school classrooms into holding centers for those suspected of carrying the viral disease. Even so, neither bedding nor basic medical equipment were available. For the most part this effort turned out to be useless.

In similar straits, Dr. Melvin Korkor, in charge of Phebe Hospital in Liberia, spoke of repeated delays in receiving much needed materials, none of which was available in the region. Many patients did not receive basic medications. Supplies of test tubes, hospital gowns, and fluids were depleted. Medical staff lacked basic safety equipment and sterile latex gloves, without which their hands were unprotected while treating patients, thus exposing these frontline health providers to the virus.[1] The end result was a high mortality rate among the care givers. Subsequently, Dr, Korkor was infected and considered himself "reborn" after surviving Ebola infection.

The lack of doctors and trained medical workers in West Africa played a role in the spread of Ebola. Liberia has only one doctor for every 100,000 people, whereas Sierra Leone has two. In comparison, the US has 245 doctors per 100,000 individuals. As hundreds of local doctors died in African communities, the Ebola outbreak escalated. Yet the WHO knew about the lack of health infrastructure in these countries, and one of their priorities should have been to plan support and enhancement of the health care network. Their responses should have been more vigorous.[1]

Failing to notify the global community about the rapid spread and danger of the Ebola outbreak was a major error. Ashish Jhna, director of the Harvard Global Health Institute stated "People at WHO were aware that there was an outbreak that was getting out of control by Spring, and yet it took until August to declare a public health emergency."[1] The Harvard Institute also accused the WHO of enabling "immense human suffering, fear, and chaos" as a result of their delayed response to the epidemic. A vivid example of poor management was the handling of early blood samples taken from infected patients to determine if they had Ebola. Some samples were shipped to laboratories where they were not examined immediately. Others sent to Paris, France, could not be tested at the recipient institution due to technical difficulties and had to be re-routed to Lyon, 250 miles away. Thus, analysis of whether an individual was infected and should be quarantined was delayed, another administrative failure.

What was the reason for the problems encountered by WHO and for its delayed actions? According to the WHO, one major obstacle was their concerns about political opposition from West African leaders. Many were cautious about taking aid because they mistrusted the source, a reflection of past exploitation by the West. Further, West African leaders feared disruption of their economies with loss of outside investments and decrease in tourism. The WHO, instead of working vigorously to resolve this difficulty, providing education, and reinforcing communication, became politically correct. When they should have announced that a major infectious outbreak from a deadly virus would hurt these countries' economies, the WHO did nothing to improve those relationships. Sensitive cultural differences made the WHO leery of disrupting any countries' feelings. Culture and politics most often trump science and reason. The WHO bowed primarily to political pressure rather than health concerns. Critics have said, and we concur, that the WHO should have understood that traditional and natural practices in the region stood in the way of effective mechanisms to contain the virus, and WHO had a moral obligation to act as educators, organize teachers, and share scientific knowledge of what the outcome would be not only to political leaders of government but most importantly to local tribal leaders.

Inadequate funds and, when available at all, poorly used expenditures were part of the problem. The leader of Doctors Without Borders, Ebola response team, Christopher Stokes, said it was 'ridiculous' that volunteers working for his charitable group were bearing the brunt of care in the worst affected countries and that international efforts will not have any effect for more than a month.[1] As a defense for not arranging to provide sufficient funding to control Ebola' destruction, Director-General Margaret Chan of the WHO explained that the WHO is not an implementation agency for outbreak response:

> "First and foremost, people need to understand WHO. WHO is the UN specialized agency in health. And we are not the first responder. You know, the government has first priority to take care of their people and provide health care. WHO is a technical agency. So, this is how we provide services. We are not like international National Government Organizations (NGOs), for example Doctors Without Borders, Red Cross, Red Crescent or local NGOs who are working on the ground to provide, you know, direct services."[1]

However, the WHO has the pulpit on the world stage to organize international efforts. In this it was negligent. WHO should have been crisp in effective decisions to fight Ebola. It was not. Instead of acting decisively, it was wishy-washy, consensus-building approach catered to political correctness. We believe that the WHO should act aggressively once the science is known during potential major health disasters to mobilize world support for disease control. Previously, they followed that kind of aggressive policy to combat the first 21st century epidemic, SARS, but that was at a different time and under different leadership.[3] A safe political bureaucracy should not be the game plan funding the WHO. In view of the lax and poor WHO effort, thought might be given to a different agency, one whose track record is rapid response, effective and efficient organization, survey, treatment and providing needing education. Such an organization with all these need virtues is Doctors without Borders.

Additional problems further hindered any effective control of Ebola' spread. Officials in many countries blocked or delayed responses to the outbreaks by denying visas to scientists, doctors, and healthcare workers who tried to cross their borders to help the victims.

The World Bank, an international agency that provides loans to developing countries, also made errors during the Ebola outbreak. Predominant was its slow response and poor cooperation with the WHO. The World Bank had opportunities early during the outbreak to meet the requests of scientists and government officials for finances to cover basic, necessary operations but chose to procrastinate. Oxfam, an international confederation of 18 NGOs working with partners in over 90 countries, criticized the World Bank for its failure to invest enough in the region's health care infrastructure. Jim Kim, president of the World Bank, admitted his institution's failures, "We should have done so many things. Healthcare systems should have been built. There should have been monitoring when the first cases were reported. There should have been an organized response."[1]

Many critics have pointed out that the delay in response to the rapidly spreading Ebola virus infection was caused, in large part, by the lack of cooperation and disagreement between the WHO and World Bank on a plan of action. Kim admitted that failure and stated, "The most important thing is to stop arguing about what is or is not possible and to get on with doing what is needed."[1]

In contrast, the African Development Bank played a large part in contributing funds to the beleaguered communities. This contribution, along with those from other NGOs, international organizations, and countries, appears in the figure below. In 2014, the African Development Bank provided a total of 223 million US dollars to Guinea, Liberia, and Sierra Leone. The bank collaborated with WHO to provide additional resources including medicines, equipment, and emergency training. In addition to the promised and paid contributions, the African Development Bank also established two new post-crises operations to lessen and prevent the instability and chaos caused by the Ebola outbreak. These operations included the establishment of an African Centre for Disease Control, and a post Ebola Livelihoods Restoration Project.[1]

An important goal of the United Nations (UN) is to provide humanitarian aid in times of famine and natural disasters. However, this time, the UN did not live up to its responsibilities. According to Doctors Without Borders, the UN had minimal impact on the epidemic regardless of their international pledges and deployments of staff. However, David Nabarro, a medical doctor who organized and led the UN mission to alleviate Ebola, disagreed, "I am absolutely certain that when we look at the history, this effort that has been put in place will have been shown to have had an impact, though I will accept that we probably won't see a reduction in the outbreak curve until the end of the year."[1] All told, Doctors Without Borders was the front-line team in the fight against Ebola despite their frustration with the lack of support in terms of action and supplies they received during the epidemic. Doctors without Borders ran most Ebola treatment facilities across the region, providing over 700 of the 1,000 beds available. The UN was not the source of front-line defenders fighting the epidemic.

The international community of nations was also deficient in the humanitarian effort it should have supplied to West Africa.[15] Instead of providing much needed medical or financial resources towards alleviating the outbreak, large and wealthy countries such as China, Russia, and Saudi Arabia barely contributed anything. In contrast, a smaller country such as Cuba and a rich country such as Sweden participated in larger, prominent, and more effective ways. The majority of donations provided came from the US AND UK. The United States funded over a third of the UN relief fund. Several banks and private philanthropists were also active contribution

Shamefully, responses from the rest of Europe and the European Union were limited and quite unsatisfactory. For example, France pledged $89.7 million; $44.85 million in direct bilateral aid and $44.85 million to multilateral institutions, a meager contribution from its $2.61 trillion economy. Northern European countries donated a significant amount more than Germany, which has one of the largest economies in Europe. Germany agreed to donate $13.37 million, contributed to supplying international aircraft and to building a field house with 300 beds in Guinea. The Netherlands has contributed the most among its regional neighbors.[1] Canada pledged over $100 million and sent supplies.

Although possessing a small economy, Cuba played a significant role in providing medical staff. Cuba sent substantial human resources in that more than 460 doctors and medical staff went to ease the crisis in West Africa. Other South American countries also donated: Brazil pledged $450,000 to the WHO along with donating five supply kits, each of which can protect 500 workers from Ebola. Chile and Columbia donated funds.[1]

To better understand contributions and commitments of countries, it is relevant to examine how much countries donated relative to their economy.

Although the US and UK pledged the most funds among all countries, some smaller countries surprisingly pledged more money relative to their GDP. Along with the UK and

US, Canada as well as Australia and Japan stand out as having contributed the most relative to their economy. Other countries such as China, Russia, Italy, France and Germany were poor donors, and why they were not more involved is unclear. The World Food Program, in particular, lashed out at Beijing's wealthy. "Where are the Chinese billionaires and their potential impact? Because this is the time that they could really have such a huge impact," said Brett Rierson, WFP representative in China.[1] However private donors and the government of China provided meager responses, considering that China is a major investor in the region of Africa most heavily infected. Although it was in China's best interest to expand their influence and potential contacts among the African countries, the government and private sector in China contributed a total of only $8.3 million to the UN main Ebola relief fund (compared to more than $200 million from the US. Of that $8.3 million, only $4.89 million came from the Chinese government. China expanded its medical staff in Sierra Leone to 50 laboratory members and promised to contribute another $34 million but was tardy in fulfilling that obligation. Beijing announced that it would donate up to $4 million to the WHO.[1]

Like governments, non-governmental organizations, and multi-national corporations, other international organizations played a smaller than expected role during the Ebola crisis. In fact, NGOs, specifically private philanthropists, and wealthy individual charities, donated more funding than many multiple national corporations. Over 60 NGOs, foundations, and charities subsidized much-needed equipment and supplies.[1] Among the major contributors were: The Bill and Melinda Gates Foundation, Oxfam, Save the Children, Paul G Allen Family Foundation, Silicon Valley Community Foundation, and the Ikea Foundation

Multinational corporations, also known as Corporate Enterprises, were slow to respond to the battle against Ebola, although they had done so quickly and generously during past calamities. Many companies that drew on natural resources in West Africa offered little to no help. For example, the cocoa industry relies heavily on West Africa. Seventy percent of the world's supply comes from this region. Yet, large multinational corporations like Nestle, Mars Chocolate, and Hershey's donated a meager $700,000 to their Cocoa Foundation to support the effort against Ebola.[1]

Even as the international community responded far less generously for the 2013-2016 Ebola epidemic then they had in the past, international organizations such as the WHO, World Bank, and UN also did too little. At the end of the day, it seems that everyone insisted something should be done, but few acted. "Nearly everyone involved in the outbreak response failed to see some fairly plain writing on the wall. A perfect storm was brewing, ready to burst open in full force", according to the internal WHO report.[1]

Since so much wrong, how can the world community plan so this infection when it happens again is better controlled and does not spread to a disaster? Put another way, "Those who fail to learn from history, are doomed to repeat it." Further, as populations in West and Central Africa increase and more humans infringe into the forest area, likely a new Ebola epidemic will occur. So, a storm is brewing. Ebola virus infections have continually occurred over the years but will another occur that involves a large population. What is needed for adequate preparations for a global warning/prepared system, and implementation of a response system?

SIX STEPS FOR DESIGNING A WORLD HEALTH RESPONSE PLAN:

First, better cooperation and communication among international agencies, governments, and NGOs are required. To accomplish this task, the development of, commitment to, and signaling of a single global institution with the responsibility for natural and environmental epidemics may be essential. Would it be more effective to create a new institution, rather than giving the authority to an existing global institution such as the CDC, WHO, or UN? The best argument for a new institution is to generate one with a single focus. The current global institutions simply have too many responsibilities and priorities. Creating a solely "non-political" and lean institution whose primary goal is for the rapid response and recovery of global and natural health disasters would eliminate the lengthy and bloated bureaucratic process so that action would be taken quickly and efficiently. This institution should also have full authority to build a reserve fund and distribute raised assets where they are most needed. The recent 2018-2020 Ebola virus outbreak in Central Africa occurred two years after the outbreak in West Africa and infected over 3,000 individuals. What lesions from the 2013-2016 were learned and corrections made? If many of the same organizational faults were made again then there is the need to evaluate the handling of the epidemic and make the needed changes.

The latter recommendation clearly requires a second step: implementation of an emergency fund. Acquiring a fund with a realistic budget, pre-pledged donations, and accumulated resources would allow immediate action. A rapid action plan would impact disease outbreak by quickly downmodulating its spread. This fund would be used for emergency preparations, recruitment of personnel, transport of staff and supplies. Routinely updating listing of doctors and health care workers, as well as plans for training populations in third-world areas where outbreaks are likely to occur must be ready. Also, necessary medicines and medical equipment should be stocked, stored safely, and available. One would have to gather international support and trust in creating a new global institution for this goal.[1] To do so, the world's sources of wealth must be convinced to fund an enterprise that manages epidemic-specific activities and to routinely allocate part of their GDP to this effort. The world is getting smaller. Infections caused by Ebola, Zika, Lassa and Severe Acute Respiratory viruses like Sars-Covid-19 are more easily transported by air flight than ever before. Thus, the threats of these epidemics are today's reality not only in countries where outbreaks occur, but in all countries engaged in global trade.[1,23,24] The current 2019-2020 Covid-19 outbreak forcefully makes this point.

The third recommendation is to prepare fully for the possible spread of viruses like Ebola and Lassa by bioterrorism. In the past (1918-1919) an influenza epidemic infected over 5% of the world's population and killed approximately 2% (over 50 million people).[25] The World Bank projected that the cost of inaction of a worldwide influenza epidemic would reduce global wealth by over $3 trillion.[26]

A fourth issue is the failure of Ebola containment. This was, in large part, caused by the lack of a universal, robust disease surveillance system. Ideally, such surveillance systems would be part of a global public health network. The ability to perform in-depth, rapid sequencing to identify the virus in question in hours or at least by a day is now available. This sequencing of individual blood samples during ongoing epidemics is now possible even in remote areas, where most outbreaks occur.[27] Surveillance helps increase effective communication among global institutions, countries, and citizens and would greatly decrease the impact of any epidemic.

In the past, and the current Covid-19 pandemic confirms self-serving politicians, government officials and flawed policies frequently caused delays that killed and continue to kill thousands; therefore, the fifth issue of reforms in global health care is to avoid bureaucratic management that prevents the speedy and worldwide release of data that forecast epidemics. The essential mandate is that, once data are obtained and verified, they are released immediately, not withheld for personal gain or credit or by countries wishing to mislead travelers and businesses.

The sixth recommendation in this World Health Plan is that essential investments should be made to train teams of doctors, medical staff, health care workers and researchers. During the 2013-2016 Ebola outbreak enormous demand for doctors, nurses, and medical staff was not matched. Training in global health should be a component of infectious disease training not only in Ebola-susceptible countries but also in the medical schools and residencies of European, American, and Asian countries. The West African countries where Ebola infection prevailed still lack doctors. The lack of basic equipment in Ebola-afflicted West Africa contributed to the large number of deaths and unsafe medical practices among health care workers. In addition, protective equipment -- uniforms, gloves and head ware -- should be readily available. The Bill and Melinda Gates Foundation suggests, "We need to invest in better disease-surveillance and laboratory-testing capacity, for normal situations and for epidemics. Routine surveillance systems should be designed in such a way that they can detect early signs of an outbreak beyond their sentinel sites and be quickly scaled up during epidemics...and the data derived from such testing need to be made public immediately. Many laboratories in developing countries have been financed by the polio-eradication campaign, so we will have to determine what capacities will be needed once that campaign is over."[28]

Finally, improved education would better ensure public understanding of how a virus spreads, the value of quarantine, and basic public health measures that could stop the spread of an ongoing epidemic or pandemic. An important lesson taught by the 2013-2016 Ebola outbreak is that the susceptible populations must be educated in what and why public health measures are needed. The local heads of countries, districts, most importantly village and national leaders, must understand how disease travels, so they can lead and guide their populations in turn. Along with these recommendations, courage, grit, and prayer should provide the format and strength to complete the goals of successful public health control of future epidemics.

Ebola's Arrival in Central Africa (2018-2020) and Its Scorecard: Turning Despair to Deliverance: Effective Anti-Viral Drugs and a Vaccine - a Road Map for COVID-19

DESPAIR

Two unresolved and pertinent questions are, first, not if but when will Ebola virus infection recur again and, second, will the outbreak be contained or spread widely as the 2013-2016 epidemic did? Since Ebola virus was initially identified in 1976 in the Central African country of the Democratic Republic of the Congo (DRC, formerly called Zaire) with 318 confirmed cases and a mortality of 88%[1] (Figure 1), eighteen of nineteen subsequent outbreaks of Ebola occurred in Central Africa. The exception was the Ebola scourge during 2013-2016 in West

Africa. The earlier Central African outbreaks caused from 425 to 6 confirmed cases with an average of 128 cases, and a mortality rate of 89% to 25% (average 63% mortality)[2] (Figure 1). By contrast the 2013-2016 episode in West Africa infected over 28,600 individuals, an increase of 222-fold over the average number of confirmed cases in Central Africa[2] (Figure 1). The mortality rate in West Africa was 40%. The same virus, Ebola-Zaire strain, was responsible for the 1976 episode, most other Central Africa outbreaks, as well as the West African plague.[2-5] Having extensive experience and evidence of what could and what did go wrong resulting in the massive, uncontrolled spread of Ebola in 2013-2016, one could ask what steps are needed by local, National, and International communities to combat and limit the spread of the next, sure to arrive Ebola outbreak (see Chapter 9). Based on historic experience with Ebola infection (Figure1), the next outbreak was likely to occur in Central Africa. The population there had/was expanding, economies had improved as did roads and highways. With increased life expectancy and finances, more vehicles were on hand to allow easier and more rapid migration from "hot spots" of Ebola to unprotected communities. Further, enhanced venturing of the population into jungles and forests for economic development and gathering of food was predictable. This set the stage for augmented contact with bats and chimpanzees, both of which carried the virus and posed a source for infecting humans.[2,6,7] Added difficulties were the civil unrest in Central Africa, especially in the DRC, where bands of migrating militias and anti-government forces raged.[8,9] Public health structure and facilities remained poor, exacerbated by mistrust in the regional and national government and western medicine. Other defects exposed in the West African 2013-2016 Ebola outbreak and in need of correction were the meager and delayed financial and health care commitment arranged through the WHO. Similarly, local, National and International agencies, non-government organizations (NGOs), and philanthropies needed greater commitment, better communication and far more efficient co-ordination than occurred in the 2013-2016 Ebola infection cycle (see Chapter 9). Will these agencies be willing and able to step into the breech for the next Ebola outbreak?

Additionally, the anti-viral drug ZMapp[10] (Chapter 5) was only serendipitously available in 2014, had not yet undergone clinical trials for safety or anti-viral effectiveness in humans. ZMapp was given to five Ebola infected individuals in 2014 and showed mixed results. Would other new anti-viral drugs be developed, and with ZMapp gone through non-human ani-mal studies with Ebola virus challenge and human safety trial? Would these anti-Ebola virus drugs be manufactured in enough quantities to be tested on humans infected with Ebola? Were protocols drawn up and approved for treatment of humans, endorsed and approved by African governments, NIH, CDC, WHO, Doctors without Borders, manufactures, etc.? Would enough health care workers be trained, physicians available, and African natives educated, ready and willing to participate in the field studies to prove or disprove the effectiveness of the anti-Ebola virus therapy?[11] Lastly, the Merck Ebola vac-cine (rVSV-ZEBOV named Ervebo) administered in Guinea during the 2013-2016 Ebola outbreak and reported to yield favorable results[12,13] (although controversial),[14] be manufactured in enough doses, and have human subject approval for clinical trials? Addressing these concerns should not and did not wait long. Indeed, these important questions and issues would be addressed within two years after the West Africa Ebola experi-ence. In 2018, Ebola again reared its head infecting a large and vulnerable population in DRC[2,15-17] (Figure 1).

In August 2018, the minister of health of DRC confirmed cases of Ebola in North Kivu province and in Ituri, likely three months after the first patient was identified. Then nearly two years later, the 25th of June 2020, the WHO declared an end of that outbreak. Confirmed cases had totaled 3,481 with 2,299 deaths, a mortality of 89%. However, circumstances during this period interfered with gathering accurate statistics. Populations were traumatized by traveling militia and other anti-government forces that targeted local clinics, killed health care workers, and attacked funeral teams as they buried the dead. Families often hid sick relatives from authorities, so neither the true numbers of Ebola infected individuals nor a final tally of deaths is known. Compounding this health crisis were a corresponding 310,000 cases of measles with 6,000 deaths, and in 2020 the outbreak of COVID-19.

The first likely Ebola case was on 30th April 2018. Two months later, clusters of acute hemorrhagic fever cases were found in Mangena village located in the Malakabo rural zone in North Kivu. It took an additional two months to confirm that the acute hemorrhagic outbreak was caused by Ebola as identified in samples sent to the Institute National de Reserche Biomedical Laboratory located in Kinshasa DRC. The DRC minister of health then notified the WHO. Within another two months after the initial outbreak, the virus spread proceeded northward to Ituri province, and by five months (September 2018) spread eastward to infect individuals in the city of Beni. From Beni, infections flowed south to involve the cities of Butembo and Katwa. These cities are commercial hubs linked to and located across from the country of Uganda by Lake Albert. During this time, the national government's handling of the outbreak improved as did the international response. DRC, WHO, and roughly 50 international partners become involved as did the dependable Doctors without Borders. About 88% of disease alerts were usually investigated within the first 24 hours, approximately 280 suspected cases were listed per day. Meanwhile, the interval from identification of a suspected clinical case to alerting health authorities of an Ebola identification was six days. Laboratory capacities of the local and national government were strengthened with the ability to identify the virus by PCR, tests to detect antibodies to Ebola virus, and sequencing of the virus genome. Despite the population's mobility, there was screening for Ebola at 80 ports of entry into the neighboring countries of Uganda, Ruanda, and South Sudan. Over 55 million screenings were done and confirmed that several individuals tested positive for Ebola had entered Uganda.[18] Approximately 75,000 Congolese crossed Lake Albert into Uganda to flee the DRC Ebola crisis.

Extensive political infighting that exploited fear and confusion before the 2018 December national election limited voting and encouraged distrust of the government leaders in charge. Opposition candidates even claimed the Ebola outbreak was drummed up to interfere with the national election. President Joseph Kabila, who reigned for eighteen years, selected his interior minister Emmanuel Ramazoni Shoday as his successor. On December 2018, the DRC Independent National Election Commission raised concerns about Ebola virus outbreaks and terrorism as a means to postponing the election in three areas in North Kivu (Beni, Beniville, Butembo) that had anti-government support. Roughly one million voters would be disenfranchised. Covering the election, writers Mo Ibrahim and Alan Doss reported "Congo's election: a defeat for democracy, a disaster for the people."

As discussed previously (Chapter 9) and below, despite the potential hazard, the WHO, likely for political reasons, failed to declare the Ebola outbreak a pandemic emergency. Although in several areas considerable improvement had been noted in epidemic control over that of the 2013-2016 Ebola outbreak, defects remained in time needed to identify patients, send specimens for analysis, receive laboratory results confirming Ebola infection, and record appropriate data. Identification of individuals in close contact with those shown to be infected with Ebola was less than 44%. Family, friends, and contacts of the sick were reluctant to be identified, indicating the need for better education and communication at the local level. Such cooperation was essential, since Ebola virus infection had never been reported before in this region of DRC. It was critical to offset the natives' distrust of not only the government but also aspects of Western medicine and health care. Typically, locals believed that controlling Ebola infections was a business decision to reward the rich and powerful in their desire to obtain land and minerals, and to sell body parts. Especially bothersome to local natives was the requirement to change traditional burial rites. So, largely uncounted numbers of such victims were buried secretly without exercising public health measure of not touching the deceased and thereby passing on the infection. Estimates are that 43% of Ebola deaths occurred outside of treatment centers and private hospitals. Delayed in communication of infectious outbreaks, failure to employ appropriate health care persona, and too little organizational funding remained. The WHO again was tardy and lax in fund raising to support the Ebola outbreak, and in controlling the potential spread of Ebola to other countries.

Accordingly, Ebola soon reached Mbandaka in the Equateur province. Forty-four Ebola infected persons, 23 died (mortality 52%). Mbandaka is a city that has a land and river connection to Kinshasa (formerly Leopoldville), a city with a population of over 11 million situated along the Congo river. Further, Mbandaka directly faces the city of Brazzaville, the capital and largest city (over 2.4 million people) of the neighboring country, Republic of the Congo. Certainly, an outbreak of Ebola in such large populations would be catastrophic. United Nations forces and escorts of armed police formed and actively tried to protect community response teams in Ebola virus infected areas.[19,20] However, their resources and complex geographic territory often limited their abilities to succeed. Irregular but frequent attacks on health care clinics and workers primarily by Islamic Fundamentalist and the so-called Allied Democratic Force continued to force several participating governments and agencies to remove their personnel for security reasons. For example, the United States removed from the area their CDC and NIH personnel.

DELIVERANCE

It was into this cauldron where Ebola virus infection re-emerged in 2018 and spread throughout relatively large populations already fraught with native unrest and suspicion. This epidemic was further augmented by roving anti-health and anti-government militias,[19,20] difficulties of delayed disease surveillance and test responses, and insufficient number of health care clinics. Geographic problems limited accessibility. A strike of health care workers also occurred. Remarkably though, nearly 3,000 health care and investigative workers both native and foreign had gathered to mount clinically controlled field trials that would define and obtain vaccination data documenting the significant inhibition of the spread of virus to uninfected individuals. Completed trials of therapeutics identified two drugs that significantly reduced the morbidity and mortality of acutely Ebola-infected individuals. These results were a testimony to the work of thousands of native health care workers recruited by the Government and Ministry of Health of DRC and international health teams. Together they registered over 250,000 individuals for field trials, tested over 220,000 samples and provided the candidate subjects needed for the vaccine and anti-viral field studies. Medical care was offered for surviving participants.

The only realistic way to test a vaccine's ability to prevent the spread of a virus from infected persons to healthy individuals is by large clinical trials. To accomplish a clinical trial of Merck's Ervebo vaccine, Doctors without Borders and the WHO personnel volunteered as the primary workers. First, it was necessary to identify acutely ill Ebola patients according to their clinical examination and obtain confirmative evidence by PCR testing that Ebola virus was the agent of infection. After measuring the amount of virus each patient carried, medical care and appropriate clinical laboratory testing proceeded. It is estimated that 35-50% of acutely ill patients, without anti-Ebola virus therapy would be saved by clinical care and replacement of lost fluids. Workers, after determining the Ebola infected individual sort direct and indirect immediate contacts of that Ebola virus infected patient. Direct or primary contacts were those individuals who were uninfected but lived with the ill patient, shared utensils/linen, and/or participated directly in the care of the sick person at least a month prior to the recorded infection. Indirect or secondary contacts were persons who had travelled with or worked with the ill patient or had contact with him/her in markets, a month before the index case infection. Before initiating the trial, all national and international institutions involved in the process must approve the Human Subjects Research procedure. To participate in the study, the method used and harm/benefit features of the vaccine or an anti-Ebola virus new drug had to be explained, understood by the recipient and then signed by those registered in the clinical trials and witnessed. Within two weeks of starting the Ervebo study, 7,500 doses of vaccine were given to primary and secondary contacts of Ebola infected individuals. The plan used for these trials is called the ring strategy, where vaccinations or primary and secondary contacts are present in a ring around the infected index case. Eventually over 300,000 individuals would be vaccinated under the ring strategy. Of the first 100,000 uninfected candidates vaccinated after 10 or more days of exposure to an Ebola virus infected person, 15 became ill but none died. Those vaccinated within the first 10 days of exposure to an Ebola virus infected patient, 56 became ill with 9 deaths, resulting in 16% mortality or 84% protection. By comparison, 61-67% mortality occurred among non-vaccinated Ebola virus infected individuals. Based on these outcomes, the WHO called the Merck vaccine effective in blocking the spread of Ebola. Wells and colleagues[21] estimated that the vaccination program in geographical area at risk reduced the level of risk for infection within that region by up to 70% if given early. However, a delay of over one week reduced the protective effect to 33-45%. The U.S. Federal Drug Administration (FDA), on December 19, 2019, approved the Merck vaccine, Ervebo, for the prevention of Ebola virus disease. This approval was a critical milestone in public health preparation, organization and response. Anna Abram, the FDA Deputy Commissioner for Policy, Legislation, and International Affairs, said "While the risk of Ebola virus disease in the U.S. remains low, the U.S. Government remains deeply committed to fighting devastating Ebola outbreaks in Africa, including the current outbreak in the Democratic Republic of the Congo. Today's approval is an important step in our continuing efforts to fight Ebola in close coordination with our partners across the U.S. Department of Health and Human Services, as well as our international partners, such as the World Health Organization. These efforts, including today's landmark approval, reflect the FDA's unwavering dedication to leveraging our expertise to facilitate the development and availability of safe and effective medical products to address urgent public health needs and fight infectious diseases, as part of our vital public health mission." Peter Marks, director of FDA's Center for Biologics Evaluation and Research added "Ebola virus disease is a rare but severe and often deadly disease that knows no borders. Vaccination is essential to help prevent outbreaks and to stop the Ebola virus from spreading when outbreaks occur. The FDA's approval of Ervebo is a major advance in helping to protect against the Zaire Ebola virus as well as advancing U.S. Government preparedness efforts. The research approach used to study the effectiveness and safety of this vaccine was precedent-setting during a public health emergency and may help create a model for future studies under similar circumstances."

What do we know about the vaccine? We know that viruses basically are made of an internal core of genes primarily required for replication and production of viral progeny and a gene that encodes for a protein on the outside surface of the virus. That glycoprotein binds to the receptor on the surface of a cell to allow virus to attach to and enter the cell. By this means virus enters the cell and infection is initiated. Ebola virus belongs to a select group of the most dangerous viruses known. Therefore, it would be difficult or impossible to use a vaccine containing the Ebola virus, per se, even after it was attenuated (weakened) because of the potential virulence for humans. The Ervebo vaccine was made at Merck & Co. under the supervision of Roger Perlmutter, Director of Research, Beth-Ann Griswold, and the company's scientists. One strategy for making a vaccine, and the one used at Merck, is to create a union of two viruses using the less human disease-causing vesicular stomatitis virus (VSV) to which just the glycoprotein of Ebola is inserted. The expressed glycoprotein gene of Ebola by itself cannot cause Ebola infection. The VSV is then used as a vehicle to transmit the glycoprotein gene into a permissive cell effectively and with minimal clinical symptoms (any symptoms would be caused by VSV). This composite virus is recorder as r (or recombinant) VSV-EBOLA GP (glycoprotein) and named Ervebo. Using this procedure there is no replication of the infectious Ebola virus, just replication of the Ebola virus glycoprotein. A potential difficulty with this type of vaccine is that replication of live and not killed Ervebo is necessary; therefore, this vaccine must be stored at -70° degrees. That requirement would be a concern especially in area/countries with limited freezers and spotty electricity to maintain the needed temperature. However, that problem was overcome in Central Africa.

The most effective vaccine would generate a protective immune response against the virus like that occurring in individuals who naturally survive the infection. Although survival tests in non-primate humans often predict of potential protective human immune response, they do not always correlate. In Ebola challenge studies of Ebola- vaccinated cynomolgus and macaque monkeys,[22,23] the generation of antibodies was necessary as were CD4 T cells that supply help to B cells to make antibody.[22] Although deletion of CD8 T cells did not impair survival of those animals vaccinated, the role for CD8 T cells was unclear. Up-regulation of markers for CD8 T cell genes (RNA analysis)[23] was noted in the CD8 T cell-deleted protected animals suggesting that the CD8 T cell deletion was incomplete. Biologic studies to show if CD8 T killing occurred were not done. Currently, no CD8 T cell data are available for the 2018-2020 Ebola outbreak. However, results for non-vaccinated immune survivors of the 2013-2016 Ebola outbreak showed that of 30 Ebola infected individuals who survived, 26 generated a robust cytotoxic T cell response in an overnight assay.[24] Others generated cytotoxic CD8 T cell response but required a longer assay, indicating these responders had a lower frequency of such cells. All 30 subjects had generated neutralizing antibodies, but such antibodies usually appear only after viruses have been purged from those individuals. Results from a study of four patients acutely infected with Ebola and then transported to the U.S. for treatment showed activation of both antibody producing cells and CD8 T cells.[25] Thus, based on these studies, it is most probable that both the humoral (antibody) and cellular (T cell) immune responses are necessary. Currently there are no data on immune responses during the first eight days of the acute Ebola infection.

Treatment of acutely infected Ebola individuals using anti-Ebola virus drugs were visited 16 months into the raging 2018-2020 outbreak. Candidates for treatment had laboratory (PCR) evidence of Ebola RNA. Volunteers to participate in the field trial were divided at random into four treatment groups. One group received ZMapp, a drug composed of three monoclonal antibodies. ZMapp had been used for a limited number of infected individuals during the 2013-2016 Ebola outbreak in West Africa (see Chapter 5). But the results were inconsistent. The second group received mAb114 (a single unique monoclonal antibody). The third group received REGN-EB3 (cocktail of three different monoclonal antibodies). The fourth and last group received the anti-viral drug remdesivir. Remdesivir is a chemical that interferes with Ebola replication in infected cells.

All these four drugs have been shown to inhibit Ebola virus infection in cultured cells and in experimental animals. However, there was no guarantee that any of these medications would be effective in humans.

All subjects enrolled in the field trial had daily clinical examinations and laboratory tests as needed. Intravenous fluid replacement was given when required as were antibiotics and anti-malaria medications. Six hundred and eighty-one patients were enrolled, and the trial was terminated after 28 days of treatment. The study was co-sponsored by the NIAID (National Institute of Allergy and Infectious Disease) of the NIH (National Institutes of Health) and carried out by an International Research Consortium (Palm Consortium Study Group) consisting of the WHO, several international financial donors, four pharmaceutical companies (ZMapp Bio, Gilead, Regeneron, Ridgeback Biotherapeutics) and Doctors without Borders. The results were recorded by an independent monitoring board. The data generated indicated significantly favorable results with two of the drugs: mAb 114 and REGN-EB3, and the trial was terminated. Monoclonal Ab114 and REGN-EB3 reduced death rate by 35% and 34%, respectively and cleared the virus from acutely infected patients. By contrast, neither ZMapp nor remdesivir purged virus from the blood, and death rates of these recipients were 49% and 53%, respectively. From that point on, all Ebola infected patients received either REGN-EB3 or mAb 114.[26,27]

When Ebola virus infection was recognized and treated early then a survival rate of about 90% was considered a realistic estimate. Dr Anthony Fauci, director of NIAID said, "They (mAb 114 and REGN-EBC) are the first drugs that a significantly sound trial has clearly shown a significant diminishing of mortality for Ebola virus infected patients. Very good news for the fight against Ebola. What this means is that we now have what looks like (two) treatments for a disease for which not long ago we really had no approach at all." Sabue Mulangu, the WHO infectious disease researcher and worker directly in the trial commented "this finding means that more than 90% of people survive if treated early." Jeremy Farrah, director of Wellcome Trust Global Health Center noted, "we won't ever get rid of Ebola but we should be able to stop these outbreaks from turning into major national and regional epidemics," while Mike Ryan head of the WHO Emergency Program commented, "The news today is fantastic. It gives us a new tool in our toolbox against Ebola, but it will not in itself stop Ebola."

Any scorecard grading the handling of the 2018-2020 Ebola virus outbreak would take note of the success in identifying and use of both an effective vaccine to limit the spread and anti-viral drugs to lessen the mortality of the devastating Ebola virus infection. This was an extraordinary and splendid feat achieved by a grand alliance of many participants who played essential roles in obtaining this breakthrough in public health and medical outcome under very difficult circumstances. Yet, in addition to very successful components, there were deficiencies noted that need attention. Implementation of appropriate corrections would ensure faster and more favorable outcomes when the next Ebola virus outbreak occurs. Adjustments would lead to better preparation to take advantage of the tools we now possess to limit the devastation caused by Ebola virus in human lives and in collapsing economies in this area of the world. The evaluation was obtained both on my assessment of the events as they occurred and insights from an experienced health care worker in the viral hemorrhagic field in Africa. In summary, the outstanding groups ahead of the curve were Doctors without Borders and NIAID. Valuable facilitators were multiple individuals from DRC health care, the WHO, pharmaceutical companies, non-government organizations, and international volunteers. Less impressive was the DRC government whose environment was often unsafe. They used the Ebola outbreak for political gain and could do better in education of their population. Similarly, the WHO's effort was mixed, although better that its performance in the 2013-2016 outbreak. In contrast to the excellence of workers on the ground, their numbers were too small for the staff far below those who stayed in Geneva. In many instances, required responses were too slow. For example, treatment sites suffered shortages of reagents, protective equipment for health care personnel, and funds to pay them. Too little control was in place to handle the migration of fleeing population from hot spots in DRC to neighboring sites and countries. Politics ruled instead of science. Overall, the WHO's impact was less helpful than Doctors Without Borders, and deficient in raising non-government and International money funds.

As a personal confession, I believe strongly in and am positive about the function of the WHO as others are.[28] I served on the WHO committee for the eradication of poliomyelitis and measles viruses, as well as on the executive board of the WHO. My experience in those years' past was a mixture of very good and dedicated people but also with a large group of in-house Geneva bureaucrats. Recently, I asked the following questions about the handling of the 2018-2020 Ebola outbreak from a dedicated non-African virus hemorrhagic expert knowledgeable in the area, as to what deficiencies uncovered in the 2013-2016 Ebola outbreak in West Africa were corrected in the recent 2018-2020 outbreak in the DRC. Below are the responses to the questions I asked:

1. Was there better cooperation and communication among international agencies (WHO, World Bank, National and International governments, NGOs [like Gates])?

   "No. Cooperation and communication was still not ideal. WHO had people on the ground but can't be said to have led the response."

2. Was there or is there a need for creation of a single global institution, non-political, lean and rapidly acting

group whose primary goal is the prevention of and recovery from Ebola epidemics, to avoid lengthy, slow, and
bloated bureaucracy?

"Yes. That would be ideal. Doctors Without Borders
(which should be supported) comes closest to this now,
but their work is very much in silo often without or in
spite of any meaningful role by governments."

3. Was an emergency fund set up to allow immediate ac-
   tion, for preparation recruitment, supplies, shipping?
   "No. but there were emergency appropriations by
   USAID, WHO and others, but not immediate."

4. Was there expansion of global investments for international health. Realizing that disease in Africa can spread
   globally?
   "NIH has expanded its emerging infectious disease
   program, which is welcome, but their commitments are
   many and resources are limited."

5. Was there a setup of surveillance systems, epidemiologic
   visits, field sequencing, or diagnostic tools?
   "No some of this is happening, but it is early and not
   systematic."

6. Was there avoidance of bureaucratic issues, rapid release
   and verification of data?
   "No."

7. Was there movement to invest in training doctors,
   public health people, health care workers not only in
   Africa but also in western countries for hemorrhagic
   fever diseases?
   "No, there are trainings but not stepped up and not
   adequate."

8. Was there improvement in facilities, education about disease so one knew what was happening and what to do by government officials, local head of districts and village leaders?

"No. Some countries are better off, particularly Nigeria and Senegal where there is strong leadership. South Africa has strong facilities built for HIV/AIDS. The continent has seen very little advancement since 2016."

So, in the end a moral lesson have we learned from these Ebola outbreaks is this. We are one people, on this planet earth. Working together we can accomplishment great things. What was achieved in the 2018-2020 outbreak of the Ebola plague in terms of a vaccine and effective anti-viral therapies is a testament to what can be done. The imagination and intelligence of humans is needed and can outplay our unfriendly infectious agents. With confidence as Ebola is now contained, we can expect COVID-19 infection to follow. Again, the poetic lines of John Donne ring and provide remembrances that were as true four hundred years ago as they were in Africa and are today in the USA.

Every man's death diminishes me,
For I am involved in mankind,
Therefore, send not to know,
For whom the bell tolls,
It tolls for thee

REFERENCES

Introduction

1   BBC Staff. "Profile: Leading Ebola Doctor Sheik Umar Khan." BBC News. Accessed July 30, 2014. http://www.bbc.com/news/world-africa-28560507
2   Fox News Staff. "Sierra Leone 'hero' Doctor's Death Exposes Slow Ebola Response." Fox News Health. August 25, 2014. Accessed May 23, 2016. http://www.foxnews.com/health/2014/08/25/sierra-leon e-hero-doctor-death-exposes-slow-ebola-response.html
3   Qiu, X. et al. Reversion of advanced Ebola virus disease in non-human primates with ZMapp. Nature 514:47-53, 2014.
4   Levs, Josh, and Jacque Wilson. "'Miraculous Day' as American Ebola Patients Reeased." CNN Health. August 21, 2014. Accessed March 3, 2016. http://www.cnn.com/2014/08/21/health/ebola-patient-release/index.html
5   "Profile: Leading Ebola Doctor Sheik Umar Khan." CNN. July 30, 2014. Accessed March 5, 2016. http://www.bbc.com/news/world-africa-28560507
6   Crowe, Kelly. "Dying Sierra Leone Dr. Sheik Umar Khan Never Told Ebola Drug Was Available." CBC News. August 18, 2014. Accessed March 6, 2016. http://www.cbc.ca/news/health/dying-sierra-leone-d r-sheik-umar-khan-never-told-ebola-drug-was-available-1.2738163
7   Ministry of Health, Democratic Republic of the Congo; WHO.

Chapter 1

1   "Peter Piot and the Ebola Outbreak in the Yambuku in 1976." LSHTM Library. October 16, 2013. Accessed April 2, 2016. http://lshtmlib. blogspot.com/2013/10/peter-piot-and-ebola-outbreak-in.html.
2   Oldstone, Michael B.A. "Hantavirus." In Viruses Plagues & History, pp. 241-246, New York, NY: Oxford University Press, 2020.
3   Oldstone, Michael B.A. "Ebola." In Viruses Plagues & History, pp. 223-246, New York, NY: Oxford University Press, 2020.
4   Gire S, Goba A, Andersen K et al. Genomic surveillance elucidates Ebola virus origin and transmission during the 2014 outbreak. Science 345, 1369-1372, 2014.

5   Kahn, J., Amarasinghe,G., Perry,D. "Filoviridae: Marburg and Ebola Viruses." In Fields Virology, D, Knipe@ P. Howley eds. 7ᵗʰ ed. 449-503, Philadelphia, PA: Lippincott Williams & Wilkins, 2020.

6   CDC. "Outbreaks Chronology: Ebola Virus Disease." Centers for Disease Control and Prevention. July 18, 2015. Accessed March 4, 2015. http://www.cdc.gov/vhf/ebola/outbreaks/history/chronology.html

7   "Tai Forest National Park - Cote Ivoire." African Natural Heritage. 2016. Accessed March 10, 2016. http://www.africannaturalheritage.org/tai-forest-national-park-cote-divoire/.

8   Report of an International Commission. "Ebola Hemorrhagic Fever in Zaire, 1976." Bulletin of the World Health Organization 56, no. 2 (1978): 271-93.

9   Heymann, David L. "Ebola: Learn from the past." Nature.com. October 9, 2014. Accessed June 15, 2016. http://www.nature.com/news/ebola-learn-from-the-past-1.16117.

10 Hildebrandt, Amber. "Ebola Outbreak: Why Liberia's Quarantine in West Point Slum Will Fail." CBC News World. August 25, 2014. Accessed March 6, 2016. http://www.cbc.ca/news/world/ebola-outbreak-why-liberia-s-quarantine-in-west-point-slum-will-fail-1.2744292.

11 Callaway, Ewen. "Hunt for Ebola's Wild Hideout Takes off as Epidemic Wanes." Nature.com. January 12, 2016. Accessed May 16, 2016. http://www.nature.com/news/hunt-for-ebola-s-wild-hideout-takes-off-as-epidemic-wanes-1.19149.

12 Leroy, Eric M., Brice Kumulungui, Xavier Pourrut, Pierre Rouquet, Alexandre Hassanin, Philippe Yaba, Andre Delicatt, Janusz T. Paweska, Jean-Paul Gonzalez, and Robert Swanepoel. "Fruit Bats as Reservoirs of Ebola Virus." Nature 438, 575-576, 2005.

13 "Ebola (Ebola Virus Disease)." Centers for Disease Control and Prevention. February 18, 2016. Accessed March 7, 2016. http://www.cdc.gov/vhf/ebola/about.html.

Chapter 2

1   "Ground Zero in Guinea: The Ebola Outbreak Smoulders – Undetected – for More than 3 Months." WHO. 2016. Accessed May 12, 2016. http://www.who.int/csr/disease/ebola/ebola-6-months/guinea/en/.

2   Quammen, David. "Insect-Eating Bat May Be Origin of Ebola Outbreak, New Study S." National Geographic. December 30, 2014. Accessed March 6, 2016. http://news.nationalgeographic.com/new

s/2014/12/141230-ebola-virus-origin-insect-bats-meliandou-reserv
oir-host/.

3   Peter Piot and the Ebola Outbreak in the Yambuku in 1976." LSHTM
    Library. October 16, 2013. Accessed April 2, 2016. http://lshtmlib.
    blogspot.com/2013/10/peter-piot-and-ebola-outbreak-in.html.

4   "Ebola (Ebola virus disease): 2014-2016 outbreak distribution in west
    Africa. https://www.cdc.gov.-vhf-2014-2016.

5   Sack, Kevin, Sheri Fink, Pam Belluck, and Adam Nossiter. "How
    Ebola Roared Back." The New York Times. December 29, 2014.
    Accessed March 7, 2016. http://www.nytimes.com/2014/12/30/health/
    how-ebola-roared-back.html?_r=0.

6   "Ebola Virus Disease in Guinea." WHO. March 23, 2014. Accessed
    April 16, 2016. http://www.afro.who.int/en/clusters-a-programmes/
    dpc/epidemic-a-pandemic-alert-and-response/outbreak-news/406
    3-ebola-hemorrhagic-fever-in-guinea.html.

7   Baize S, Pannetier D, Oestereich L, el al. Emergence of Zaire
    Ebola Virus Disease in Guinea." New England Journal of Medicine
    371,1418-1425, 2014.

8   Geisbert TW, Pushko P, Anderson K, Smith J, Davis KJ, Jahrling PB.
    "Evaluation in Nonhuman Primates of Vaccines." Emerg Infect Dis,
    8(5):503-7. May 2002. Accessed June 11, 2016. http://www.ncbi.nlm.
    nih.gov/pubmed/11996686.

9   Gire, S Goba A, Andersen K, et al. Genomic surveillance of Ebola
    virus origin and transmission during the 2014 outbreak Science
    345:1369-1372, 2014.

10 Reuters,   Thomson.   "Bats   Likely   Carry   Ebola   to
    Humans, but May Also Carry Cure - Technology &
    Science - CBC News." CBCnews. November 03, 2014. Accessed April
    15, 2016. http://www.cbc.ca/news/technology/bats-likely-carry-ebola-t
    o-humans-but-may-also-carry-cure-1.2821851.

11 Vidal, John. "Ebola: Research Team Says Migrating Fruit Bats
    Responsible for Outbreak." The Guardian. August 23, 2014. Accessed
    June 10, 2016. https://www.theguardian.com/society/2014/aug/23/
    ebola-outbreak-blamed-on-fruit-bats-africa.

12 Vogel, Gretchen. "Bat-filled Tree May Have Been Ground Zero
    for the Ebola Epidemic." Science and AAAS. December 30, 2014.
    Accessed March 9, 2016. http://www.sciencemag.org/news/2014/12/
    bat-filled-tree-may-have-been-ground-zero-ebola-epidemic.

13 "New WHO Safe and Dignified Burial Protocol- Key to Reducing
    Ebola Transmission." World Health Organization. November 7,

2014. Accessed March 10, 2016. http://www.who.int/mediacentre/news/notes/2014/ebola-burial-protocol/en/.

14 Schnirring, Lisa. "Probe of Ebola Burial Practices Pinpoints Risks, Triggers Change." CIDRAP. January 13, 2015. Accessed March 15, 2016. http://www.cidrap.umn.edu/news-perspective/2015/01/probe-ebola-burial-practices-pinpoints-risks-triggers-changes.

15 Fletcher, Pascal. "As Ebola Stalks West Africa, Medics Fight Mistrust, Hostility." Reuters. July 13, 2014. Accessed March 15, 2016. http://www.reuters.com/article/health-ebola-westafrica-idUSL6N0PO0V220140713.

16 The Editors of Encyclopedia Britannica. "African Religions." Encyclopedia Britannica. Accessed April 22, 2016. http://www.britannica.com/topic/African-religions.

17 "Ebola Cremation Ruling Prompts Secret Burials in Liberia." The Guardian. October 24, 2014. http://www.theguardian.com/world/2014/oct/24/ebola-cremation-ruling-secret-burials-liberia.

18 Charlton, Corey. "Bribery Breaks out in Battle against Ebola: Liberian Victims' Families Paying Corrupt Retrieval Teams to Keep Bodies so They Can Give Them Traditional Burials." Daily Mail. October 14, 2014. Accessed April 29, 2016. http://www.dailymail.co.uk/news/article-2791911/bribery-breaks-battle-against-ebola-liberian-victims-families-paying-corrupt-retrieval-teams-bodies-traditional-burials.html.

19 "Sierra Leone: A Traditional Healer and a Funeral." World Health Organization. 2016. Accessed April 12, 2016. http://www.who.int/csr/disease/ebola/ebola-6-months/sierra-leone/en/.

20 Oldstone. M.B.A.: "Ebola." In Viruses, Plagues and History, pp. 223-240, New York, NY Oxford University Press, 2020.

Chapter 3

1 "Kenema Government Hospital." Viral Hemorrhagic Fever Consortium. Accessed June 17, 2016. http://vhfc.org/consortium/partners/kgh.

2 Radoshitzky,S.,Buchmeier, M., de la Torre, J.C Arenaviridae: The viruses and their replication. In: Fields Virology, 7th Edition. D.M. Knipe @ P.M. Howley, Eds.,784-809 Lippincott, Williams & Wilkins, Philadelphia, 2020.

3 Ogbu O, Ajuluchukwu E, Uneke CJ. "Lassa fever in West African sub-region: an overview". Journal of vector borne diseases 44 (1): 1–11, 2007.

4   Oldstone, M.B.A. "Lassa Fever." In: Viruses, Plagues, & History, pp. 215-222, Oxford University Press, New York, NY 2020.

5   "2014 Ebola Outbreak in West Africa - Case Counts." Centers for Disease Control and Prevention. April 14, 2016. Accessed June 18, 2016. http://www.cdc.gov/vhf/ebola/outbreaks/2014-west-africa/case-counts.html.25

6   Preston, Richard. The Hot Zone: The Terrifying True Story of the Origins of the Ebola Virus. Anchor Books,1995.

7   McCormick J., King, I.,Webb,P.A. et al. "Lassa fever." The New England Journal of Medicine, 314, 20-26, 1986.

8   McCormicK J., Fisher-Hoch H. Lassa fever in Arenaviruses I. The epidemiology, molecular and cell biology. Curr. Topics Microbiol. Immunol. 262. M.B.A. Oldstone, Ed., Springer-Verlag, Berlin, 2002.

9   Jang, Se Young. "The Causes of the Sierra Leone Civil War." E-International Relations. October 25, 2012. Accessed April 18, 2016. http://www.e-ir.info/2012/10/25/the-causes-of-the-sierra-leone-civil-war-underlying-grievances-and-the-role-of-the-revolutionary-united-front/.

10 "Sierra Leone Rebels Forcefully Recruit Child Soldiers." Human Rights Watch. June 31, 2000. https://www.hrw.org/news/2000/05/31/sierra-leone-rebels-forcefully-recruit-child-soldiers.

11 Catalanello,R. "Q@A with Tulane Researchers on Front Line of Ebola Outbreak. "NOLA. com. August 28,2014. http://www.nola.com/health/index.ssf/2014/08/qa_with_tulane_researcher_who.html

12 http://broadfoundationreport.org/portfolio/stories/science/pardis-sabeti-broad-institute-voices-from-the-frontlines-of-an-epidemic/.

13 "2014 Ebola Outbreak in West Africa - Case Counts." Centers for Disease Control and Prevention. April 14, 2016. Accessed June 18, 2016. http://www.cdc.gov/vhf/ebola/outbreaks/2014-west-africa/case-counts.html.

14 "Ebola Virus Disease Outbreak." World Health Organization. 2016. Accessed June 18, 2016. http://www.who.int/csr/disease/ebola/en/.

15 "Sierra Leonean Government Honors VHFC Team Members." Viral Hemorrhagic Fever Consortium. January 24, 2016. Accessed April 12, 2016. http://www.vhfc.org/media/news/sierra-leonean-government-honors-vhfc-team-members.

16 Schieffelin, John S., Jeffrey G. Shaffer, and Augustine Goba. "Clinical Illness and Outcomes in Patients with Ebola in Sierra Leone." The New England Journal of Medicine 371, 2092-2100, 2014.

17 "Profile: Leading Ebola Doctor Sheik Ulmar Kahn." BBC News. July 30,2014.hppt://www.bbc.com/news/world-africa-28560507.

18 Sakabe, S., Sullivan, B., Harnett, J. el al Analysis of CD8 T response during the 2013-2016 Ebola epidemic in West Africa. PNAS 115, 7578-7586, 2018.

19 Wong, G. et.al, Mers,Sars and Ebola: the role of super-spreaders in infectious disease Cell Host@ Microbe 18, 398-401, 2015.

20 Gire S, Goba A, Andersen K, et al. Genomic Surveillance Elucidates Ebola Virus Origin and Transmission during the 2014 Outbreak Science 345, 1369-1372, 2014.

21 Park D, Dudas G, Wohl S, et al. Ebola Epidemiology transmission and Evolution during several months in Sierra Leone Cell 161, 1516-1526, 2015.

22 Oldstone M.B.A. "Ebola." In Viruses, Plagues and History, pp. 223-240, Oxford University Press, New York, NY, 2020.

Chapter 4

1   Oldstone, Michael B.A. "Lassa Fever." In Viruses Plagues & History, pp. 215-222, New York, NY: Oxford University Press, 2020.

2   Radoshitzky S., Buchmeier, M., de la Torre J.C. Arenaviridae: The viruses and their replication. In: Fields Virology, 7th Edition. D.M. Knipe and P.M. Howley, eds., pp. 784-809, Lippincott, Williams & Wilkins, Philadelphia, 2020.

3   Sakabe, S., Sullivan, B., Hartnett, J., et al Analysis of CD8 T response during the 2013-2016 Ebola epidemic in West Africa. PNAS 115, 7578-7586, 2018.

4   Oldstone, Michael B.A. Identification and validation of novel human T cell epitopes in Lassa fever and Ebola. NIH Contract HHSN272201400048C under BAA-NIAID-DAIT-NIHAI2013167 "Large scale T cell epitope discovery" 2014-2019.

5   "Head Doctor Fighting Ebola Outbreak in Sierra Leone Contracts the Deadly Virus." Reuters News. July 23, 2014. Accessed June 4, 2016. http://www.telegraph.co.uk/news/worldnews/africaandindian-ocean/sierraleone/10986310/Head-doctor-fighting-Ebola-outbreak-in-Sierra-Leone-contracts-the-deadly-virus.html.

6   Hammer, Joshua. "My Nurses Are Dead, and I Don't Know I'm Already Infected." Matter. January 12, 2015. Accessed April 15, 2016. https://medium.com/matter/did-sierra-leones-hero-doctor-have-to-die-1c1de004941e#.fcqm5t8a4.

7   "Dr. Sheik Humar Khan." Viral Hemorrhagic Fever Consortium. Accessed May 16, 2016. http://vhfc.org/consortium/people/humarr-khan.

8   Sanchez, Nick. "Sheik Umar Khan, Sierra Leone's Top Ebola Doc, Catches the Disease." NewsMax. July 24, 2014. Accessed May 24, 2016. http://www.newsmax.com/TheWire/sheik-umar-khan-ebola-doctor/2014/07/24/id/584621/.

9   Oldstone, M.B.A. Virus neutralization and virus-induced immune complex disease. Prog. Med. Virol. 19:84-119, 1975.

10   Qui X, Wong G, Audet J et al., Reversion of advanced Ebola virus disease in non-human primates with ZMapp. Nature 514:47-53, 2014.

11   Omonzejele P.F. Ethical challenges posed by the Ebola virus epidemic in West Africa. J. Bioeth. Inq. 11:417-420, 2014.

12   Wilson, Jacque. "Ebola Doctor in Sierra Leone Dies." CNN. July 31, 2014. Accessed April 15, 2016. http://www.cnn.com/2014/07/29/health/ebola-doctor-dies/index.html.

Chapter 5

1   Oldstone. M.B.A. "Human Immunodeficientcy Virus (HIV): AIDS the Current Plague." In Viruses, Plagues, & History, pp. 295-330, Oxford University Press, New York, NY 2020.

2   Oldstone, M.B.A. "Hepatitis Viruses: Oysters, Blood Transfusions and Cancer." In Viruses, Plagues and History, pp. 187-202, Oxford University Press, New York, NY, 2020.

3   Warren T, Jordon R, Lo M, et al. Therapeutic efficacy of the small molecule GS-5734 against Ebola virus in rhesus monkeys Nature 531:381-383, 2016.

4   Oldstone. M.B.A. Molecular mimicry: Infection inducing autoimmune disease. Curr. Topics Microbiol. Immunol., Springer-Verlag, Heidelberg, 2005.

5   Heeney J, Ebola: Hidden reservoirs. Nature 527:453-455, 2015.

6   Chughtau A, Barnes M, Macintyre C . Persistence of Ebola virus in various body fluids during convalescence: evidence and implications for disease transmission and control. Epidemiol. Infect. 144:1652-1660, 2016.

7   Sakabe.S, Sullivan, B., Harnett, J.et al Analysis of CD8 T response during the 2013-2016 Ebola epidemic in West Africa PNAS 115:7578-7586, 2018.

8   van Griensven J, and the Ebola Outbreak Epidemiology Team. Evaluation of convalescent plasma for Ebola disease in Guinea. N. Engl. J. Med. 374:33-42, 2016.

9   Corti D, Misasi, J, Mulangu, S Protective Monoclonal antibody against lethal Ebola virus. Science 351:1339-1342, 2016.

10 Patel, A. It takes a mature antibody to treat Ebola infection. Science Direct 9 Jan 2019.

11 Bornholdt Z, Turner H, et al., Isolation of Potential Neutralizing Antibodies from a survivor of the 2014 Ebola outbreak: Science 351:1078-1083, 2016.

12 Zeitlin L, Geisbert J, Deer D, et al., Monoclonal antibody therapy for Junin virus infection: PNAS 113:4458-4463, 2016.

13 Gautam R, et al., Broadly neutralizing antibodies: magic bullets against HIV: Nature 533:105-109, 2016.

14 McElroy, A.K. et al. Human Ebola infection results in substantial: immune activation: PNAS 112:4719-4724, 2015.

15 Qiu X, Wong G, Audet J. et al. Reversal of advanced Ebola virus disease in non-human primates Nature 514:47-53, 2014.

16 Omonzejele P.F. Ethical challenges posed by the Ebola virus epidemic in West Africa. J. Bioeth. Inq. 11:417-420, 2014.

Chapter 6

1   Mueller, Katherine. "Turning to Traditional Healers to Help Stop the Ebola Outbreak in Sierra Leone." IFRC. July 31, 2014. Accessed March 12, 2016. http://www.ifrc.org/en/news-and-media/news-stories/africa/sierra-leone/turning-to-traditional-healers-to-help-stop-the-ebola-outbreak-in-sierra-leone-66529/.

2   Kuhn J, Andersen K, Baize S et al. Nomenclature-and database-compatible names for the two Ebola virus variants that emerged in Guinea and the Democratic Republic of the Congo in 2014. Viruses 6:60-99, 2014.

3   Gire S, Goba A, Andersen K, et al. Genomic surveillance elucidates Ebola virus origin and transmission during the 2014 outbreak. Science 345:1369-1372, 2014.

4   "NIAID Role in Ebola and Marburg Research." NIH. February 26, 2016. Accessed April 14, 2016. http://www.niaid.nih.gov/topics/ebolaMarburg/research/Pages/default.aspx.

5   "The People of Tulane Cancer Center Research." Tulane University - School of Medicine - Robert F Garry. Accessed April 16, 2016. http://tulane.edu/som/cancer/research/people/robert-f-garry.cfm.

6   Catalanello, R. "Tulane Researchers Race to Develop Rapid Ebola Finger-prick Test." NOLA.com. October 13, 2014. Accessed April 3, 2016. http://www.nola.com/health/index.ssf/2014/10/tulane_researchers_race_to_dev.html.

7 Oldstone, M.B.A. "Ebola." In Viruses, Plagues and History, pp. 223-240, Oxford University Press, New York, NY, 2020.

8 "2014 Ebola Outbreak in West Africa - Outbreak Distribution Map." Centers for Disease Control and Prevention. March 17, 2016. Accessed June 14, 2016. http://www.cdc.gov/vhf/ebola/outbreaks/2014-west-africa/distribution-map.html.

9 "Conflict Diamonds." Amnesty International USA. Accessed June 1, 2016. http://www.amnestyusa.org/our-work/issues/business-and-human-rights/oil-gas-and-mining-industries/conflict-diamonds.

10 McCormick J., King,I.J., Webb, P.A. et al. Lassa Fever. N Eng J Med :314 20-26, 1986.

11 "In Memory of Dr. Sheik Humar Khan." Africa Centre Of Excellence for Genomics of Infectious Diseases:10 August 7, 2014. Accessed April 20, 2016. http://acegid.org/index.php?active=page.

12 "Viral Hemorrhagic Fever Consortium." Viral Hemorrhagic Fever Consortium. Accessed June 20, 2016. http://www.vhfc.org/.

13 "Africa Centre Of Excellence for Genomics of Infectious Diseases." Africa Centre Of Excellence for Genomics of Infectious Diseases. 2016. Accessed June 20, 2016. http://acegid.org/.

14 "Consortium." H3Africa Human Heredity & Health in Africa. Accessed June 20, 2016. http://www.h3africa.org/consortium.

15 Yi-Gang Tong, Wei-Feng Shi, Di Liu, Long Liang, Xiao-Chen Bo, Jun Liu, Hong-Guang Ren, Hang Fan, Ming Ni, Yang Sun, Yuan Jin, Yue Teng, Zhen Li, David Kargbo, et al. Genetic Diversity and Evolutionary Dynamics of Ebola Virus in Sierra Leone. Nature 524, 93-96, 2015.

16 Schieffelin, J., Shaffer, J., Goba,A., et al. "Clinical Illness and Outcomes in Patients with Ebola in Sierra Leone." The New England Journal of Medicine 371, 2092-2100, 2014.

17 Kuhn,J., Amarasinghe, G., Perry, D. in Filoviridae: Marburg and Ebola Viruses, in: Fields Virology, 449-503 7th Ed. Philadelphia, PA: Lippincott Williams & Wilkins, 2002.

18 "Press Release - VHFC Researchers Publish Key Findings on the 2014 Ebola Outbreak." Viral Hemorrhagic Fever Consortium. August 28, 2014. Accessed June 20, 2016. http://www.vhfc.org/media/news/press-release-vhfc-researchers-publish-key-findings-2014-ebola-outbreak.

Chapter 7

1 "Kenema Government Hospital." Viral Hemorrhagic Fever Consortium. Accessed May 20, 2016. http://vhfc.org/consortium/partners/kgh.

2   Oskin, Becky. "Awardee Profile - Pardis Sabeti." Burroughs Wellcome Fund. 2014. Accessed June 20, 2016. http://www.bwfund. org/newsroom/awardee-profiles/awardee-profile-pardis-sabeti.

3   "Pardis Sabeti Computational Geneticist." National Geographic. 2016. Accessed June 5, 2016. http://www.nationalgeographic.com/ explorers/bios/pardis-sabeti/.

4   Cao,W., Henry, M.D., Borrow, P Yamada,H.,Elder,J.,Ravkov,E.,Nichol, S.,Compans, R. Campbell,K., M.B.A. Oldstone. Identification of alpha-dystroglycan as a receptor for lymphocytic choriomeningitis virus and Lassa fever virus. Science 282, 2079-81,1998.

5   Kunz,S., Sevilla,N.,McGavern,D.,Campbell,K.,Oldstone, M.B.A. Molecular analysis of the interaction of LCMV with its cellular receptor alpha-dystroglycan. J Cell Biol:155,301-10, 2001.

6   "ACEGID." Africa Centre Of Excellence for Genomics of Infectious Diseases 2016. Accessed March 20, 2016. http://acegid.org/index. php?active=page.

7   "Iranian Scientist Is One of Time's Persons of the Year." Iranian Scientist Is One of Time's Persons of the Year. December 26, 2014. Accessed June 20, 2016. http://iran-times.com/iranian-scientist-is-on e-of-times-persons-of-the-year/.

8   Mnookin, Seth. "Pardis Sabeti, the Rollerblading Rock Star Scientist of Harvard." Smithsonian. December 2012. Accessed March 2, 2016. http://www.smithsonianmag.com/science-nature/pardis-sabeti-th e-rollerblading-rock-star-scientist-of-harvard-135532753/.

9   Gire S, Goba A, Andersen, K, et al. Genomic surveillance elucidates Ebola virus origin and transmission during the 2014 outbreak. Science 345:1369-1372, 2014.

10 Baize S, Pannetier D, Oestereich L, et al. Emergence of Zaire Ebola virus disease in Guinea. N Eng J Med 371,1418-1425, 2014.

11 Simon, Scott. "Borders Close As Ebola Spreads In West Africa." Borders Close As Ebola Spreads In West Africa. August 23, 2014. Accessed June 20, 2016. http://www.npr.org/2014/08/23/342652013/ borders-close-as-ebola-spreads-in-west-africa.

12 Holmes E.C, Dudas G, Rambaut A, Andersen K.G. The evolution of Ebola virus: insights from the 2013-2016 epidemic. Nature 538:193-200, 2016.

13 Dodds, Kieran. "Fruit Bats: Africa's Greatest Mammal Migration." Discover Wildlife. July 24, 2010. Accessed March 4, 2016. http://www. discoverwildlife.com/animals/fruit-bats-africas-greatest-mamma l-migration.

14 James, Davy. "Tracking Fruit Bats May Identify Regions at Greatest Risk for Ebola Epidemic." Pharmacy Times. September 11, 2014. Accessed June 20, 2016. http://www.pharmacytimes.com/news/Tracking-Fruit-Bats-May-Identify-Regions-at-Greatest-Risk-for-Ebola-Epidemic.

Chapter 8

1 Amadou S, Amy Copley A. "Understanding the Economic Effects of the 2014 Ebola Outbreak in West Africa." The Brookings Institution. October 01, 2014. Accessed June 20, 2016. http://www.brookings.edu/blogs/africa-in-focus/posts/2014/10/01-ebola-outbreak-west-africa-sy-copley.
2 Kelly J.D. Making diagnostic centers a priority for Ebola crisis. Nature 513:145, 2014.
3 Geewax M. "World Bank Says Ebola Could Inflict Enormous Economic Losses." NPR. October 8, 2014. Accessed March 12, 2016. http://www.npr.org/sections/thetwo-way/2014/10/08/354599549/world-bank-says-ebola-could-inflict-enormous-economic-losses.
4 Jallanzo A. "Ebola: Economic Impact Could Be Devastating." World Bank. August 2014. Accessed April 22, 2016. http://www.worldbank.org/en/region/afr/publication/ebola-economic-analysis-ebola-long-term-economic-impact-could-be-devastating.
5 Hamilton R. "Ebola Crisis: The Economic Impact." BBC News. August 21, 2014. Accessed June 13, 2016. http://www.bbc.com/news/business-28865434.
6 "Ebola Hurts More Than the Sick: World Bank." NBC News. January 12, 2015. Accessed June 20, 2016. http://www.nbcnews.com/storyline/ebola-virus-outbreak/ebola-hurts-more-sick-world-bank-n284421.
7 Odutayo A. "The Ebola Virus Disease: Problems, Consequences, Causes, and Recommendations." E-International Relations. April 22, 2015. Accessed June 20, 2016. http://www.e-ir.info/2015/04/22/the-ebola-virus-disease-problems-consequences-causes-and-recommendations/.
8 "Kenya Airways to Suspend Flights to Freetown, Monrovia Due to Ebola." Reuters. August 16, 2014. Accessed May 13, 2016. http://www.reuters.com/article/us-health-ebola-kenya-airways-idUSKBN0GG0F520140816.
9 Neate R. "Mining Company at Centre of Fight against Ebola in Sierra Leone Goes Bust." The Guardian. October 16, 2014. Accessed

June 13, 2016. http://www.theguardian.com/world/2014/oct/16/londo
n-mining-fight-ebola-sierra-leone-goes-bust.

10 "The Socio-Economic Impacts of Ebola in Liberia." World Bank.
November 19, 2014. http://www.worldbank.org/content/dam/
Worldbank/document/Poverty documents/Socio-Economic Impact
of Ebola on Households in Liberia (final).pdf.

11 11. "The Economic Impact of the 2014 Ebola Epidemic: Short and
Medium Term Estimates for West Africa." World Bank. October
8, 2014. Accessed June 13, 2016. http://www.worldbank.org/en/re-
gion/afr/publication/the-economic-impact-of-the-2014-ebola-epide
mic-short-and-medium-term-estimates-for-west-africa.

12 "UN: Nearly $1 Billion Needed to Combat Ebola Outbreak." UN
News Center. September 16, 2014. Accessed June 13, 2016. http://
www.un.org/apps/news/story.asp?NewsID=48728#.VxmRU7_Vuho.

13 Freeman C. "Cuban Doctors Take Leading Role in Fighting Ebola."
The Telegraph. January 29, 2015. Accessed June 13, 2016. http://
www.telegraph.co.uk/news/worldnews/ebola/11375422/Cuban-doctor
s-take-leading-role-in-fighting-Ebola.html.

14 "Ebola's Economic Impact." The Economist. September 03, 2014.
http://www.economist.com/blogs/baobab/2014/09/costs-pandemic.

15 Gallagher J. "Ebola Response Lethally Inadequate, Says MSF." World in
Struggle. September 2, 2014. Accessed May 13, 2016. http://worldinstrug-
gle.blogspot.com/2014/09/west-africa-ebola-plague-caused-by-imf.html.

16 "Harmonizing Policies to Transform the Trading Environment."
Assessing Regional Integration in Africa VI (October 03, 2013).
Accessed May 22, 2016. doi:10.18356/5d7bf72c-en.

17 "Ebola Hampering Household Economies across Liberia and Sierra
Leone." World Bank. January 12, 2015. Accessed May 13, 2016.
http://www.worldbank.org/en/news/press-release/2015/01/12/ebol
a-hampering-household-economies-liberia-sierra-leone.

18 Mjamba K. "Cameroon Closes Border with Nigeria over Ebola." This
Is Africa. August 18, 2016. Accessed June 13, 2016. http://thisisafrica.
me/cameroon-closes-border-nigeria-ebola/.

19 Jallanzo A. "Ebola: Economic Impact Could Be Devastating." World
Bank. August 2014. Accessed April 22, 2016. http://www.worldbank.
org/en/region/afr/publication/ebola-economic-analysis-ebola-lon
g-term-economic-impact-could-be-devastating.

20 Oldstone, M.B.A. "Severe Acute Respiratory Syndrome (SARS): The
first pandemic of the 21st century, Middle East Respiratory Syndrome
(MERS) and 2019-2020 outbreak of COVID-19 (2019-nCoV)." In

Viruses, Plagues, & History, pp. 247-260, Oxford University Press, New York, NY, 2020.

Chapter 9

1   McSpadden K. "WHO Acknowledges Failings of Ebola Response." Time. Time, 20 Apr. 2015. Web. 21 June 2016.

2   "World Health Organization Admits It Failed in Handling Ebola." NY Daily News. April 20, 2015. Accessed June 21, 2016. http://www. nydailynews.com/life-style/health/world-health-organization-admit s-failed-handling-ebola-article-1.2191334.

3   Oldstone, M.B.A. "Severe Acute Respiratory Syndrome (SARS): The first pandemic of the twenty-first century. Middle East Respiratory Syndrome (MERS) and 2019-2020 outbreak of Covid-19 (2019-nCOV)." In Viruses, Plagues, & History, pp. 247-260, New York, NY, 2020.

4   "WHO 'failed to Alert' Global Community about Ebola Outbreak Allowing Virus to Spread Further – Panel." RT International. November 23, 2015. Accessed June 21, 2016. https://www.rt.com/ne ws/323113-ebola-outbreak-who-failure/.

5   Goldberg E. "Ebola Aid Workers Shocked by WHO's 'Amateurism' In Response To Outbreak." The Huffington Post. October 05, 2014. Accessed June 21, 2016. http://www.huffingtonpost.com/2014/10/06/ who-poor-response-ebola_n_5933866.html.

6   Hinshaw D. "Ebola Virus: For Want of Gloves, Doctors Die." WSJ. August 16, 2014. Accessed June 21, 2016. http://www.wsj.com/articles/ ebola-doctors-with-no-rubber-gloves-1408142137.

7   Duff M. "Ebola Takes Big Toll on Already Poor Health Care." Ebola Takes Big Toll on Already Poor Health Care. August 30, 2014. Accessed June 21, 2016. http://www.redding.com/news/ebola-takes-bi g-toll-on-already-poor-health-care-ep-585823658-362256141.html.

8   Colen B. D. "An Indictment of Ebola Response." Harvard Gazette. November 22, 2015. Accessed June 21, 2016. http://news.harvard. edu/gazette/story/2015/11/an-indictment-of-ebola-response/.

9   "Ebola Crisis: No Impact from Pledges of Help, MSF Says." BBC News. October 17, 2014. Accessed June 21, 2016. http://www.bbc.com/ news/world-africa-29656417.

10 Fink S. "W.H.O. Leader Describes the Agency's Ebola Operations." The New York Times. September 4, 2014. Accessed June 21, 2016. http://www.nytimes.com/2014/09/04/world/africa/who-leade r-describes-the-agencys-ebola-operations.html.

11 Elliott L. "Ebola Crisis: Global Response Has 'failed Miserably', Says World Bank Chief." The Guardian. October 09, 2014. Accessed June 21, 2016. http://www.theguardian.com/world/2014/oct/08/ebola-crisi s-world-bank-president-jim-kim-failure.

12 "Global 'failure' to Grip Ebola Crisis Criticised by World Bank President | World News |." NNWnet National News Wire. October 08, 2014. Accessed June 21, 2016. http://nnw.net/global-failure-to-gri p-ebola-crisis-criticised-by-world-bank-president-world-news/.

13 "Ebola." African Development Bank Group. 2006. Accessed June 21, 2016. http://www.afdb.org/en/topics-and-sectors/topics/ebola/.

14 "Ebola Crisis: UN Envoy Rejects Criticism of Agency's Response." BBC News. October 18, 2014. Accessed June 21, 2016. http://www. bbc.com/news/world-africa-29672179.

15 "Action Taken by the Netherlands and the International Community to Tackle Ebola." Information from the Government of The Netherlands. Accessed June 21, 2016. https://www.government.nl/ topics/ebola/contents/action-taken-by-the-netherlands-and-the-int ernational-community-to-tackle-ebola.

16 Szklarz E. "Latin American Health Officials Prepare To Fight Ebola." Diálogo. October 16, 2014. Accessed June 21, 2016. http:// dialogo-americas.com/en_GB/articles/rmisa/features/2014/10/16/ feature-01?source=most_viewed.

17 Rajagopalan M. "China's Companies, Billionaires Must Step Up To Fight Ebola: WFP." Business Insider. October 20, 2014. Accessed June 21, 2016. http://www.businessinsider.com/r-chinas-companies- billionaires-must-step-up-to-fight-ebola-wfp-2014-10.

18 Sanchez R. "What Countries Have Pledged to Fight Ebola... and How Much They've Paid into the Fund." The Telegraph. October 22, 2014. Accessed June 21, 2016. http://www.telegraph.co.uk/ news/worldnews/ebola/11179135/What-countries-have-pledge d-to-fight-Ebola...-and-how-much-theyve-paid-into-the-fund. html.

19 "Non-Governmental Organizations Responding to Ebola." USAID Center for International Disaster Information CIDI. 2015. Accessed June 21, 2016. http://www.cidi.org/ebola-ngos/#.V0yr_4-cGrM.

20 Rooney B. "UN Asks $1 Billion for Ebola, Gets $14 Million so Far." CNNMoney. October 21, 2014. Accessed June 21, 2016. http://money. cnn.com/2014/10/17/news/un-ebola-funding/index.html.

21 Cheng M. "Ebola Outbreak: WHO Admits It Botched Early Attempt to Stop Disease." CBC news. October 17, 2014. Accessed June 21,

2016. http://www.cbc.ca/news/world/ebola-outbreak-who-admits-it-bo tched-early-attempt-to-stop-disease-1.2802432.

22   Rull M, Ilona KickbuscIe I, Lauer H, "International Development Policy Revue Internationale De Politique De Développement." Policy Debate. June 2, 2015. Accessed June 21, 2016. https://poldev.revues.org/2178#tocto2n3.

23   Gates B. "The Next Epidemic Lessons from Ebola — NEJM." New England Journal of Medicine. April 15, 2015. Accessed June 21, 2016. http://www.nejm.org/doi/full/10.1056/NEJMp1502918.

24   Piot P., Soka M. Spencer, J. Emergent threats: lessons learnt from Ebola. Int Health 11, 334-337, 2019.

25   Oldstone, M.B.A. "Influenza virus, the plague that will continue to return." In Viruses, Plagues, & History, pp. 355-388, Oxford University Press, New York, NY, 2020.

26   The World Bank. Pandemic risk and One Health. October 23, 2013 http://www.worldbank.org/en/topic/health/brief/pandemic-risk-one-health.

27   Holmer E., Gytis D., Rambaut A, Andersen K. "The evolution of Ebola virus: Insights from the 2013-2016 epidemic." Nature 538:193-200, 2016

28   Levy, Y., Lane,C., Piot,P., et al. Prevention of Ebola virus disease through vaccination: where we are in 2018. Lancet 392, 787-790, 2018.

Chapter 10

1   "Peter Piot and the Ebola Outbreak in the Yambuku in 1976." LSHTM Library. October 16, 2013. Accessed April 2, 2016. http://lshtmlib.blogspot.com/2013/10/peter-piot-and-ebola-outbreak-in.html.

2   Oldstone, Michael B.A. "Ebola." In Viruses Plagues & History, pp. 223-246, Oxford University Press, New York, NY, 2020.

3   Baize S, Pannetier D, Oestereich L, el al. "Emergence of Zaire Ebola Virus Disease in Guinea." New England Journal of Medicine 371,1418-1425, 2014.

4   Gire S, Goba A, Andersen K, et al. Genomic surveillance of Ebola virus origin and transmission during the 2014 outbreak. Science 345, 1369-1372, 2014.

5   Basler CF. Portrait of a killer: genome of the 2014 EBOV outbreak strain. Cell Host Microbe 16, 419-421, 2014.

6   Reuters, Thomson. "Bats Likely Carry Ebola to Humans, but May Also Carry Cure-Technology&Science-CBCNews."CBCnews.November03, 2014. Accessed April 15, 2016. http://www.cbc.ca/news/technology/bat s-likely-carry-ebola-to-humans-but-may-also-carry-cure-1.2821851.

7   James, Davy. "Tracking Fruit Bats May Identify Regions at Greatest Risk for Ebola Epidemic." Pharmacy Times. September 11, 2014. Accessed June 20, 2016. http://www.pharmacytimes.com/news/ Tracking-Fruit-Bats-May-Identify-Regions-at-Greatest-Risk-for-Ebola-Epidemic.

8   Ebola health workers killed and injured by rebel attack in Congo, Guardian 28 Nov 2019 https://www.the guardian com/ global-development.

9   What will it take to finally end Congo Ebola outbreak https://kpbs. org/news/2020/jan/09.

10 Qiu X, Wong G, Audet J. et al. Reversal of advanced Ebola virus disease in non-human primates. Nature 514:47-53, 2014.

11 Omonzejele P.F. Ethical challenges posed by the Ebola virus epi-demic in West Africa. J. Bioeth. Inq. 11:417-420, 2014.

12 Henao-Restrepo A., Camachi A, Longini, M. Efficiency and ef-fectiveness of a r-VSV-vectored vaccine in preventing Ebola dis-ease: final results from the Guinea ring vaccination, open-label, cluster-randomized trial. Lancet 389, 505-518, 2017.

13 Levy Y. Lane C. Piot P. et al. Prevention of Ebola virus disease through vaccination: where we are in 2018. Lancet 392, 787-790, 2018.

14 Metzer W, Vivas-Martinez S. Questionable efficiency of the r-VSV-ZEBOV Ebola vaccine. Lancet 391, 1021, 2018.

15 Kalenga M, Moeti A, Sparrow A, et al. The ongoing Ebola epidemic in Democratic Republic of Congo 2018-2019. N Eng J Med 381,373-383, 2019.

16 Steinhauses G. Congo declares world's second-worse Ebola outbreak over. WSJ 26 June 2020 https://www.wsj.com/congo-declares-world-second-worse ebola-outbreak-over-115930932088.

17 Lewnard J. Ebola virus disease: 11323 deaths later, how far have we come? Science 392, 189-190, 2018.

18 Eustachewich L. Deadly Ebola outbreak spreads from Congo to Uganda. NY Post, 12 June 2019 https://nypost.com/2019/06/12/deadl y-ebola-outbreak-spreads-from congo-to-uganda/.

19 Baruyo N, Steers J. Deadly Congo attacks hurt efforts to stem Ebola crises. WSJ, 26 September 2019, A20.

20 teers J, Steinhauser G. Militant attacks worsen a growing Ebola outbreak. WSJ 15 April 2019.

21 Wells C, Pandey A, Paria A. Ebola vaccination in the Democratic Republic of the Congo. PNAS 116, 10178-10183, 2019.

22 Marzi A, Engelmann F, Feldmann F, et al. Antibodies are necessary for rVSV/ZEBOV-GP-mediated protection against lethal Ebola virus challenge in nonhuman primates. PNAS 110, 1893-1898, 2013.

23 Menicucci A, Sureshchandra S, Marzi A, Feldmann H, Messaoudi I. Transcriptomic analysis reveals a previously unknown role for CD8 T cells in rVSV-EBOV mediated protection. Sci Rep 7:919. DOI:10.1038/S41598-017-01032-8, 2017.

24 Sakabe S, Sullivan B, Harnett, J. et al. Analysis of CD8 T response during the 2013-2016 Ebola epidemic in West Africa. PNAS:115 7578-7586, 2018.

25 McElroy, A.K. et al. Human Ebola infection results in substantial: immune activation. PNAS 112:4719-4724, 2015.

26 Kupferschmidt K. Successful Ebola treatments promise to tame outbreak. Science 365, 628-629, 2019.

27 Zarocostas J. Hope for the Ebola outbreak in DR Congo. Lancet 395, 773, 2020.

28 Bloom B, Farmer P, Rubin E. WHO's next-the United States and the World Health Organization. N Eng J Med 383, 676-677, 2020.

INDEX

DRC (Democratic Republic of
Congo). *See* Democratic
Republic of the Congo
(DRC) (formerly Zaire)

E

Ebola
biology and pathogenesis of
as not completely un-
derstood, 10
carriers of. *See* bats;
chimpanzees
Central Africa outbreaks of.
See Central Africa
diagnosing of first case in
Sierra Leone. *See also*
Sierra Leone
diagnostic tests for detection
of. *See* diagnostic tests
differences with Covid-19,
xiii–xiv
difficulties in identification
of, 8–9
doubts that it exists, 67
electron micrograph drawing
of, 10*f*
first identified infection of,
1, 48
first recorded case of, 3
genetic variability of, 74
genomic analysis of, 44, 70–
71, 73, 74–75, 76–77,
81–82, 83
host of in the wild as uncertain, 30, 86
incidence of as compared to
Lassa, 26–27
infections and deaths as a
result of single index
case, 4

Kikwit outbreak…chapter 1
Kinshassa outbreak…chap-
ter 1
Kivu outbreak, 3
lessons learned from initial
outbreak of, 5–6
list of outbreaks of, 10*f*
Meliandow outbreak …chapter 2
mortality rate, xiii–xiv, 2
naming of, 1
natural reservoir of infection
for, 12–13
as negative-strand RNA virus, 12
origin of, xxiv
possibility of super viral
spreader, 35
results of genome sequencing
of, 36
as RNA virus, 11
role of in unraveling economy
of West Africa, 87–96
severity of epidemic as causing many non-African
countries concern about
exposure, 92–93
shared traits with Covid-19,
xiii
spread of/transmission of, xiv,
xvi, xxiv, 2, 3–4, 5, 7,
9, 12–13, 17, 18, 20–21,
23, 24, 28, 37, 73–74,
75, 81, 82, 83, 89, 92,
96, 97, 98, 99, 100, 101,
102, 113, 115, 118
survival rate when recognized
and treated early, 123
symptoms of, 3, 5, 28, 29, 35

tests to help identify etiologic agent responsible for outbreak of, 17–18

varied response to, 35

West Africa outbreaks of. *See* West Africa

world as unprepared for outbreak of, xvi

Ebola Makona, 54

Ebola Reston, xiv

Ebola-Taï Forest, 85–86

Ebola-Zaire, 2, 3, 14, 15, 18–19, 20, 84–85, 86, 113, 120

education efforts, 7, 8, 20–21, 33, 36, 67, 96, 111, 116

ELWA Hospital (Liberia), 63, 66

Emory University School of Medicine, Ebola survivors as transported to, 61–62

Ervebo (Merck Ebola vaccine), 114, 118–121

ethics, regarding use of ZMapp, 51, 52–68

European countries, assistance from, 92, 106, 107

Evans, David, 91

F

Farrah, Jeremy, 124

Fauci, Anthony, 123

Feldmann, Heinz, 45

filoviruses

Ebola virus as belonging to family of, 9

ZMapp's effectiveness against, 54

fluids, as only early reliable therapy for Ebola, xxii, 49, 52

Fonnie, Mballu, xxi, 24, 37, 38, 44, 48

foreign investments, Ebola's impacts on, 94–95

Formenty, Pierre, 21

Frame, John, 27

Friscia, Fabio, 67

funding. *See also* international assistance

as inadequate, 103

for surveillance, reduction in, 8

funerals. *See* dead bodies

G

Garry, Robert (Bob)

on antibody response, 59

as associated with Tulane Medical School, xxiii, xxiv, 32, 33, 44, 46, 47

background of, 71

communication with Sheik Khan by, 52

as director of International Center of Infectious Diseases Research, 73

on health care workers contracting Ebola, 38–39

as one of founders of VHFC, 73

as one of three major players involved with Ebola at KGH, xvi, 78, 80

personal and professional relationship with Sheik Khan, 75, 76

photo of, **40**

as pleading for help from international community, 36

as pressuring for Sheik Khan to get treatment, 65

Institute of Tropical Medicine,
assistance from, 8
interferons (IFNs), 35, 56, 57, 83
international assistance. *See
also specific countries and
organizations*
appeal for in Ebola outbreaks,
36–37
commitment of as overall insufficient and tardy, 96,
97, 108
as deficient in humanitarian
effort during Ebola out-
break, 105–106
UN's estimate of need for to
restrict further out-
breaks, 92
West African natives as having lack of trust in, 67
International Monetary Fund,
assistance from, 92
isolation
of exposed persons, 7
of infected persons, 5, 6, 23,
29, 32, 33, 47, 70

J

Jhna, Ashish, 102

K

Kailahun treatment center, xxi–
xxii, xxiii, 48, 49, 51, 63,
64, 65
Kamara, Fatima, 48
Katsiaficas, Bob, 42
Kelley, J. Daniel, 87–89
Kenema Government Hospital
(KGH) (Sierra Leone)

as changing priority from
Lassa virus to Ebola
treatment, 34, 43,
47, 72
described, 25–26
first Ebola-infected patient
arrives at (March 2014),
34, 69
first incidence of Ebola virus
infection at (2014), 23
LASV/Lassa program at, 18,
25, 26, 31–33, 45, 46,
72, 73
monument dedicated to
health care workers
who died in fight
against Ebola, **40**, 45
number of sick individuals
coming to, 37
patients treated by Sheik
Khan at, xxiii
photo of, **39**
Sheik Khan as head of,
xxi, 24
shifting of Lassa virus project
to, 31–33
success of care at, 100
as treating first identified
Ebola infection, 48
viral hemorrhagic fever
(VHF) ward at, 73
Kentucky Bio-Processing, 50,
64, 68
Khan, Sahid, 45
Khan, Sheik Humar/Umar
as afraid of dying from
Ebola, 47
background of, 45–47
communication with Garry
by, 52

Blood Diamonds War in, 72
civil war in, 29–31, 72
doctors in, 101
Ebola outbreaks in, xxiv, 2, 3,
    23, 24, 34, 36, 43, 54,
    73–74, 75–76, 80, 81,
    82–83, 85, 88, 98, 99
Ebola's role in unraveling
    economy of, 89–96
first incidence of Ebola virus
    infection in (2014),
    23–24, 33, 69, 70, 73,
    82, 83
Lassa fever in, xviii, 27, 30,
    33, 43, 72
Ministry of Health and
    Sanitation, 26
Silicon Valley Community
    Foundation, assistance
    from, 107
Sirleaf, Ellen Johnson, 68
smallpox, eradication of, 55
South American, assistance
    from, 106
Stokes, Christopher, 103
Sullivan, Brian, 44
surveillance programs, 4–5, 8–9,
    26, 33, 34, 96, 101, 110, 111,
    118, 126

T

T cells, 35, 44, 56–57, 58, 59–60,
    62, 83, 84, 121–122
Taï Forest (Ivory Coast) Ebola vi-
    rus strain, 2, 13–14, 82, 85
Tandala Mission Hospital, Ebola
    outbreak, 6
Thomas, D.W., 85
tourism, impacts on from Ebola's
    presence, 94

trade restrictions, use of, 93
travel restrictions, use of, 93, 95
treatments
    anti-viral drugs/antiviral
        therapies. *See* anti-vi-
        ral drugs/antiviral
        therapies
    fluids as, xxii, 49, 52
    for human viral diseases, for-
        mulation of, 53–61
    at Kailahun treatment center.
        See Kailahun treatment
        center
    at Kenema Government
        Hospital (KGH). *See*
        Kenema Government
        Hospital (KGH) (Sierra
        Leone)
    Lassa virus treatment center,
        18, 25, 26, 31–33, 45,
        46, 72, 73
    as provided by Doctors
        Without Borders.
        See Doctors Without
        Borders (Médecins
        Sans Frontières [MSF])
    for Sheik Khan as debated,
        51, 62, 63–66
    ZMapp. *See* ZMapp
Tucker, Veronica, 48
Tulane University School of
    Medicine
    Garry's association with, xxiii,
        xxiv, 32, 33, 44, 46, 47
    KGH Lassa unit in partner-
        ship with, 32
    as principal partner with
        Mano River Union
        Lassa Fever Network
        program, 32

Turner, Jeffrey D., 64

U

United Kingdom (UK), assistance from, 106
United Nations (UN)
  commitment of as over-all insufficient and tardy, 108
  failure of in communications among other international organizations, 97–98
  as not living up to its responsibilities during Ebola outbreak, 105
United States Centers for Disease Control (CDC)
  assistance from, 4, 8–9, 26, 27, 33, 63, 71
  field station in Sierra Leone moved to Guinea, 30–31
United States Communicable Disease Center, xxii
United States (US)
  assistance from, 92, 106
  shift of financial assistance for Ebola to Zika, 76
University of Texas Medical School (Galveston), 30
U.S. Department of Health and Human Services, as partner in Ebola fight, 120
U.S. Food and Drug Administration (FDA)
  approval of Merck vaccine by, 119–120
  authorization of Ebola rapid diagnostic test by, 72

V

vaccines
  benefits of, 55
  for Ebola, xv, xxiii, 52, 61, 114
  field trials of, 118–119
  role of, 58
vesicular stomatitis virus (VSV), 121
Viral Hemorrhagic Fever Consortium (VHFC), 18, 25–26, 32, 37, 38, 73–74, 78, 79, 80
viral hemorrhagic fever (VHF) ward, at Kenema Government Hospital (KGH), 73
viruses
  arenaviruses, 30, 54
  coronaviruses (SARS), 54
  filoviruses, 9, 54
  naming of, 1–2
  RNA viruses. See RNA viruses
  vesicular stomatitis virus (VSV), 121
Voice of America, on impact of Ebola on investor confidence, 94

W

Wellcome Trust, assistance from, 73
West Africa. See also Guinea; Liberia; Sierra Leone
  Ebola outbreaks in, xxi–xxiii, xxiv, xxv, 9, 13, 15, 18, 19f, 73, 84, 85, 112–113
  Ebola's role in unraveling economy of, 87–96
  migration within as easy, 13

political leaders of as fearing disruption of economics, 102

Wine, Laura, 27–28

World Bank
assistance from, 44, 73, 92
commitment of as overall insufficient and tardy, 108
on cost of inaction of worldwide influenza epidemic, 110
on economic effects of Ebola on West Africa, 87, 91–92, 94
errors made by during Ebola outbreak, 104
failure of in communications among other international organizations, 97–98, 104

World Food Program, on lack of assistance from Beijing's wealthy, 107

World Health Organization (WHO)
assistance from, xxii, 7, 26, 32, 38, 120, 124–125
authorization of Ebola rapid diagnostic test by, 72
author's confidence in, 125
clarification of role of, 103
commitment of as overall insufficient and tardy, 96, 97, 98–99, 100, 101, 102, 103–104, 108, 117
as concerned about political opposition from West African leaders, 102–103

on Ebola infections from burials of deceased Ebola patients, 21
on effectiveness of Merck vaccine, 119–120
as endorsing use of ZMapp, 68
as failing to declare Ebola outbreak as pandemic emergency, 116
handling of Ebola as compared to handling of prior epidemics, 98, 99, 104
notification of, 17
reporting end of Ebola epidemic (2016), 76

world health response plan, steps for designing of, 108–111

Writebol, Nancy, xxii, 63, 66

Y

Yambuku, Zaire, as where Ebola was first identified, 1, 3–4
Yambuku Mission Hospital, Ebola outbreak (1976), 3–4

Z

Zaire (now Democratic Republic of Congo, DRC)
Ebola-Zaire strain. *See* Ebola-Zaire
Yambuku as site where Ebola first identified, 1, 3–4

ZMapp, xxii, xxiii, 49, 50–51, 52, 62–65, 68, 114, 122–123

ZMapp Bio, 123

www.ingramcontent.com/pod-product-compliance
Lightning Source LLC
Chambersburg PA
CBHW021407210526
45463CB00001B/259